Eat
Your
Ice
Cream

Which Country Has the World's Best Health Care?

Prescription for the Future:
The Twelve Transformational Practices
of Highly Effective Medical Organizations

Reinventing American Health Care:
How the Affordable Care Act Will Improve Our
Terribly Complex, Blatantly Unjust, Outrageously
Expensive, Grossly Inefficient, Error Prone System

Brothers Emanuel:
A Memoir of an American Family

Healthcare, Guaranteed: A Simple, Secure Solution for America

No Margin, No Mission:
Health Care Organizations and the Quest for Ethical Excellence
(with Steven D. Pearson and James Sabin)

The Ends of Human Life: Medical Ethics in a Liberal Polity

Eat
Your
Ice
Cream

Six Simple Rules for a Long and Healthy Life

Ezekiel J. Emanuel, MD, PhD

W. W. NORTON & COMPANY
Independent Publishers Since 1923

For information about permission to reproduce selections from this book, write to
Permissions, W. W. Norton & Company, Inc., 500 Fifth Avenue, New York, NY 10110

For information about special discounts for bulk purchases, please contact
W. W. Norton Special Sales at specialsales@wwnorton.com or 800-233-4830

Manufacturing by Lakeside Book Company
Book design by Chris Welch
Production manager: Julia Druskin

Library of Congress Control Number: 2025945547

ISBN 978-1-324-11753-7

W. W. Norton & Company, Inc., 500 Fifth Avenue, New York, NY 10110
www.wwnorton.com

W. W. Norton & Company Ltd., 15 Carlisle Street, London W1D 3BS

Authorized EU representative: EAS, Mustamäe tee 50, 10621 Tallinn, Estonia

1 0 9 8 7 6 5 4 3 2

HR 01 06 2026 1019

To the memory of Benjamin Emanuel

My father, who modeled and thus taught me how to

Be curious

Speak my mind without fear

Be social

Care about people less fortunate than myself

Walk fast

Be financially frugal (aka a cheapskate)

Drive poorly

And, hopefully, not be a schmuck

Contents

Eat
Your
Ice
Cream

Introduction

"**A** glass of wine a day is supposed to be good for you, right?" The woman lifted her glass of red wine as if toasting a bride and groom. Before I could answer, she took a long gulp. Her tone was simultaneously coy and inquisitive, as if she were genuinely interested in the answer but worried that I might bat the drink out of her hand.

She knew I was a physician who had spent much of my career evaluating ways to help Americans live healthier lives. Over the years, I helped to write and pass the Affordable Care Act, which expanded health care access for millions of Americans, and I was part of the team that created the new food plate to replace the food pyramid. Questions like hers had become a common refrain at receptions, dinner parties, and other social gatherings. Even casual conversations about family or politics would often morph into medical consultations about what to eat or not eat, what exercises to do or avoid, or what health fads to follow or ignore.

Before I could respond, the man beside her interjected. He

had foresworn drinking since having COVID because alcohol didn't taste good anymore. Taking a sip of his alcohol-free gin and tonic, he elaborated: "I've lost a few pounds. I have more energy. I sleep better. I just feel better."

Who was right? They looked to me to adjudicate.

"Alcohol is one of the most confusing and divisive issues in wellness," I said. "Every study seems to come to a different conclusion." They looked at me imploringly, as if each hoped I'd take their side.

"Drinking is not really beneficial to your health," I said. Alcohol has a lot of calories—about 65 per ounce—with few health benefits and some serious downsides, especially for younger people. If you're talking about very moderate amounts, like three or four glasses of wine a week, it might be harmless, but any more than that can get you into real trouble. None of the reports of the so-called 'French paradox'—the idea that drinking red wine explains the low rate of coronary artery disease in France despite a decadent diet—have ever panned out.

"But everything has trade-offs," I continued. "There's plenty of evidence that time with friends is good for you, so if you have an occasional drink with friends, it probably evens out. Just don't binge drink, drink alone, or drink to drown your sorrows. Those things are definitely not good for you."

I paused, unsure whether what I'd say next would change their perspective. But I wanted them to know that their question wasn't the most important one. I concluded with the same bluntness that I give my family, friends, and even my students:

"Remember the first rule of life: *We're all going to die.* You can waste all your time trying to extend your life by a few minutes, obsessing over scores of adjustments to your diet or exercise routines, or you can follow six straightforward, smart wellness behaviors and make the time you have healthier and more meaningful."

Both of my conversants audibly exhaled. Each considered their alcohol drinking habits vindicated. But they were also curious about what else they should be doing, besides the usual advice to eat well, exercise, and sleep. Before launching into my wellness shpiel, I lifted my glass of water for a three-way toast: "To your health!"

Every second we live can never be recovered. Time goes in only one direction. The time we have is finite. We know that at some point our bodies and brains will slow, break down, and ultimately fail. It is natural. This reality motivates us to want to build lives that are as healthy, functional, and as fulfilling as possible. We naturally want to know what we can do to postpone our inevitable fate—and maximize the chances of not just living more years, but living those years with vigor. As Thoreau eloquently summarized, most of us want to "live deep and suck out all the marrow of life."

Anyone looking for advice on wellness and longevity confronts a tsunami of books, newspaper articles, podcasts, newsletters, and videos from an enormous range of sources: scientific experts, medical practitioners, health systems, journalists, patients, influencers, gurus, quacks. Traditional media offer loads of good advice, often in responsibly edited and well-sourced sections dedicated to "wellness." But the sheer amount of it can be difficult to keep up with, and sometimes the guidance can be downright contradictory.

For anyone wading through the torrent of health and longevity advice online, it can be difficult to know who to trust. The so-called "must dos" online range from the medically unproven to the wildly impractical to suggestions so absurd they leave doctors like me baffled—testicle tanning, teen blood transfusions, vaginal steaming, "rucking" hikes with a back-pack full of weights. Information is coming at us from a fire-hose, increasingly spewed by hucksters and self-proclaimed sages who have amassed millions of social media followers (and dollars) by promising supposed miracle treatments using medical-sounding language. It's no wonder so many people are confused and frustrated.

Shouting to be heard over it all are real physicians and health experts offering sound but sometimes conflicting advice. All of it together can swamp even those who are most assiduous about their health. Dozens of books on health and longevity have appeared in just the last few years, filled with well-intentioned and scientifically accurate information. But too often they fall into the trap of chasing novelty instead of efficacy and end up touting treatments and regimens that are unproven or with marginal returns at best.

Then there is the steady stream of profiles on tech bil-lionaires joylessly devoting themselves to maximizing their lifespan. One of my business school students told me how her "wellness coach" recommended all sorts of questionable pre-scriptions, like eating 200 grams of meat a day. (Don't ask me why a perfectly healthy twentysomething student who isn't training for a marathon or Ironman needs a wellness coach.) And then there is the entrepreneur attempting to defy death with his daily regimen of 100 pills, cold plunges, infrared lights, and a daily serving of "nutty pudding"—a mix of chia seeds, macadamia nuts, and berries. Nutty is right.

With so much health and wellness advice out there, it can be nearly impossible to differentiate the valid, reliable, and effective from the speculative, deceptive, and just plain stu-pid. Even when the advice is scientifically sound, it's often extraneous, misrepresented, or misused. For example, one wellness book ventures into the basic biology of molecular pathways, like the mTOR pathway for cell survival, to explain why you should take rapamycin to improve longevity. Indeed, studies have shown rapamycin extends the lifespan of mice, worms, flies, and yeast. But you are not a mouse, worm, fly, or yeast. While some studies have suggested that rapamycin for humans may mitigate the impact of aging-related immune and cardiovascular diseases, there is no evidence that it impacts human lifespans.

This extrapolation of laboratory findings parallels the story of resveratrol, the "magic" compound in grapes and red wine that was supposed to explain the French paradox. Yes, resveratrol improved longevity in mice. But, do you have a tail and whiskers? Scientists have been experimenting on mice since the early 20th century, and while this work has led to many breakthroughs, findings in mice often fail to extend to humans. As an oncologist, I know that researchers have cured hundreds of thousands of mice with cancer using experimental chemotherapy agents, only to have the drugs fail when administered to people with cancer. Unfortunately, there's no evidence that resveratrol or rapamycin improves human lifespans. Ultimately, the biology lesson and the "health advice" is a waste of people's time.

What so many of these talking heads have in common—legitimate experts, well-meaning journalists, and kooks alike—is how costly their recommendations are. Financially, for sure, but also costs in mental energy and time that steal from activites which give life meaning. With the mountain of advice out there, it is practically a full-time job to determine whether the information on rapamycin is *accurate*, not to mention if it is *worth taking*.

Overall, the wellness industrial complex promises us more time to enjoy in the future—but sure is demanding a lot of time right now. It takes a *ton* of time and attention to pore through a 400-page book, much less a whole library of them. And what about the zillions of posts, videos, and articles about the latest new supplement, superfood, or exercise that supposedly can lengthen your life? Add that to the time spent trying to figure out what is real versus what is a fad. Or based on some microbes in a petri dish or a study of worms. Or worse yet, based on no evidence at all. Then budget more time to methodically organize your schedule to incorporate the latest exercise tweak or diet advice. . . . Congratulations: You have now *lost* that added time the gurus promised you. And you've lost it in the prime of your life.

Of course, if your whole focus is on quantity of years rather than quality, this work could be worth it. Some "longevity experts" seem to see things that way. As one popular author says, "Our only goal is to live longer and live better—to outlive." Our *only* goal? Life is not a competition where the gold medal goes to the oldest! Our goal should *not* be to "outlive" as many people as possible. Instead, the goal should be to live a healthy and fulfilling life. Wellness is just a means to that end, not the end in itself.

In fact, we already live longer than almost any Americans before us. Life expectancy on the eve of the Civil War was 39.4 years, and by the start of the 20th century it had increased to just 48.2 years. Today, even with the problems of COVID and deaths related to opioids, suicide, and the like, life expectancy in the United States has reached 78.6 years. That is the average. My own research shows that the longest-lived 20% of Americans have an average lifespan of 93 years. And the longest-lived 40% of Americans have an average lifespan of over 88 years.

If Americans are already living long lives, why the obsession with wellness? Wellness was launched into mainstream America in 1979 with a *60 Minutes* segment in which the legendary journalist Mike Wallace declared that wellness is "a word you don't hear every day." His broadcast, seen by millions of Americans, helped increase public awareness and inspire a national pursuit. Soon new companies fed the growing demand, launching products to sell everything from supplements to fitness facilities to retreat centers to You-Tube channels.

It seems that upswings in wellness obsessions or lifestyle modifications seem to emerge when there is a collective sense that the world has spun out of control. When we find ourselves unable to resist, deter, or influence the bad things that befall us and our families, we begin to look for things we *can* control. We have so many political, economic, and social changes in our lives today that may be turbocharging this wellness obsession. Globalization and the deconstruction of community and country, an addictive media system that runs on algorithms we don't understand and can't escape, the unpredictability of climate change, Gilded Age–level inequality, and the worry that generative AI will control rather than be controlled by humanity. These are just a few of the problems confronting us. We feel vulnerable, anxious, and powerless—at the mercy of forces beyond our reach. So we embrace what we can control: our own wellness.

The massive wellness wave reached a fever pitch in 2025 when Dr. Casey Means, a prolific wellness influencer, was named as the US surgeon general. Dr. Means's book *Good Energy* is a bestseller and she regularly posts on Instagram, where she has more than 700,000 followers. She has used her platform to promote "mitochondrial health" gummies, algae-laden "energy bits," and vitamins she described as her "immunity stack." As *The Atlantic* put it, "Her rise is, in many ways, emblematic of modern internet wellness culture writ large: If you're articulate and confident and can convincingly recite

what seems like academic evidence, you can become famous—
and perhaps even be named surgeon general."

Of course, just because the wellness movement is driven
by a desire for control does not mean trying to improve your
health is bad or unimportant. But most of the wellness advice
out there manages to be both too complicated and too simplistic. Too complicated because wellness is not new. The essence
of wellness—the six wellness practices—is age-old wisdom.
The ancient Greeks, Chinese, and Indians knew about most
of it. Even the teachings of Hippocrates 2,500 years ago advo-
cated for good diet and exercise as the way to health: "If we
could give every individual the right amount of nourishment
and exercise, not too little and not too much, we would have
found the safest way to health." At about the same time, Aristotle devoted considerable ink in his work *Nicomachean Ethics* to the importance of close friends in pursuing a healthy,
fulfilling, virtuous life. The modern advice has unfortunately
strayed from these foundations of health.

Despite fixating on complexities, the advice out there also
remains overly simplistic—or at least incomplete. Most well-
known writers on wellness today emphasize one of three
physical components of wellness and longevity: eating, exercise, and sleep. These are all vital to living a healthy life,
but they are only half the story. The *social and psychological* components to wellness are even more important. Risk
management, friendship and social interactions, and mental
engagement have a measurably greater impact on your wellness than diet, exercise, and sleep.

There is no reason to make wellness an obsession to which
we devote oodles of hours every day. You don't want—or need—a
wellness data dump. Most people just need the bottom line—
straightforward, evidence-based dos and don'ts for the health

information that really matters. Because wellness is simple, this book is simple. It focuses on the six fundamental wellness behaviors that yield the maximum benefits with the least work:

1. Don't be a schmuck—avoid self-destructive risks
2. Talk to people—cultivate family, friends, and other social relations
3. Expand your mind—stay mentally sharp
4. Eat your ice cream—consume healthy food and drink
5. Move it!—exercise well and regularly
6. Sleep like a baby—get the rest you need

This list is short, manageable, and effective. Nobody needs an elaborate how-to guide with speculation about minor adjustments that might—or might not—add a few minutes to your life. Instead, this book aims to succinctly communicate expert recommendations on the behaviors that are important to living a healthy life. It is a distillation of the evidence to simplify doing the right thing.

The six wellness behaviors are short and simple for another reason. We have immediate and worthy demands for our time, attention, and money: loving our partners and caring for our friends, tending to and playing with our children or grandchildren or, hopefully, great grandchildren, having a productive and satisfying work life. We also have an interest in improving our neighborhoods, schools, and society in general and in being active in our churches, mosques, and synagogues. Then there are the hobbies and other activities we find fulfilling: gardening, making jam or bread, throwing a pot or knitting a scarf, painting or taking photographs, going to the ball game, theater, or museum, fishing or hiking a mountain trail, or curling up to read a mystery or watch a movie. There's a lot to be said for living fully and being present, not constantly monitoring our activity tracker or feeling guilty for not achieving every wellness goal.

My goal is to make wellness a part of the fabric of everyday life. To incorporate the main wellness behaviors as you go about your daily activities, not squeeze your life around a boundless list of wellness tasks. The wellness rules should become an invisible part of your lifestyle, sustained by habit so that they don't require mental focus or irritating drudgery.

You'll notice that there is nothing here about happiness or stress. That is because, as Eleanor Roosevelt wisely said, "Happiness is not a goal . . . it's a by-product of a life well lived." Stress, too, is a by-product of life. Following the simple guidelines here will help reduce the bad kind of stress, the kind that tends to be chronic, long term, and arising from situations we feel we cannot control—a bad job or a toxic relationship, for example. Chronic stress is the essence of anti-wellness. It can lead to long-term inflammation, make you susceptible to infections, impair your brain function, induce depression and hopelessness, and ultimately lead to premature aging. And do you know one thing that stresses out people who care about their health? Thinking about every dietary and exercise choice as if it's a life-or-death decision!

In the famous Blue Zones of the world, inhabitants routinely live to 90 or even 100 years old, remain cognitively intact, and experience few physical ailments. The people in Okinawa, Japan, Loma Linda, California, Sardinia, Italy, and the other Blue Zones are positive outliers, and they don't go around obsessed with making constant adjustments in what they eat, taking supplements, pounding the pavement, and monitoring their steps, heart rate, blood glucose, and minutes of sleep. They just live rich, healthy lives without consciously trying to maximize wellness and longevity.

The fact is, on average, people in the Blue Zones live longer and healthier lives than almost all other people on the planet. They do so by adopting lifestyle choices that are *accessible, easy,* and *impactful*—such as balanced meals, natural activity, and regular socialization—and building those things seamlessly into their daily schedules. It is not a matter of willpower or extreme sacrifice. People in Blue Zones simply focus on the things that enrich their lives with meaning and connection. They are implementing the wellness and longevity recommendations unconsciously and innately.

We can't all live in such places, but it's easy to adopt time-tested and scientifically proven behaviors to live a long, healthy, and fulfilling life. In that regard, this book is an extension of what I have tried to do my entire professional life: improve Americans' health. There are no secret treatments or exclusive wellness regimens here. This is a guide for everyone, not just those who can afford to spend a lot of money or time on their health. And I am not selling a supplement, elixir of life, or magical water from the fountain of youth Ponce de León died trying to find in Florida in 1521. Nor am I offering a very expensive battery of diagnostic tests or trademarked diet or patented exercise equipment or personalized app or spa stay. Using everything I've learned from a career in public health and health care, I will provide a concise, clear, and authoritative synopsis of what health experts know works best to bring you the biggest health benefits—without extraneous, speculative, or absurd additions.

Change is hard. After all, if the only thing standing between you and perfect health was being told to stop drinking soda and join a running club, we'd all be immortal by now. But change is not impossible. The key is to ensure that your regular schedule promotes wellness without turning yourself into a hamster on a wheel. And without making you feel shamed or stressed for failing to do more.

Willpower is an essential resource on the road to wellness. But it diminishes with repeated use. If relied on over and over, your willpower will fatigue and become depleted, making it harder to make good wellness choices. How, then, can we make changes to our routines without exhausting our willpower?

I am not a big fan of motivational mantras. They mostly strike me as corny and not very enlightening. But every so often one of them can summarize a complex idea pretty well. To that end, I have modified one of life coach and motivational speaker Bernard Burchard's graphics about the process to adopt a new wellness behavior. The four steps progress from (1) the motivation to adopt a wellness activity to (2) the initiation of the activity to (3) repetition of the activity so that eventually (4) it becomes a habit or routine part of who you are.

This mantra makes clear that you shouldn't fall for offerings like "5 days to happier, healthier eating" or "4 exercises that work immediately." They are the wellness equivalent of snake oil. For a wellness behavior to be sustainable, you have to put in the repetitions and remember that nothing worthwhile or enduring works immediately.

Willpower is critical at two points: going from the *intention* to *initiation* of the wellness behavior; and, most importantly, *repeating* the behavior enough to make it a habit. The intention-to-initiation barrier is relatively minimal. Reading this book, you already have the motivation to adopt wellness behaviors. The repetition barrier is much higher—but it's not insurmountable.

Each New Year's, millions of people around the world resolve to stop drinking, lose weight, limit sugary treats and desserts, cease smoking, or adopt any number of virtuous activities. It is called Dry January for a reason. Unfortunately, long before the end of the month, most have given up and reverted back to sipping a scotch, guzzling soda, and avoiding the gym. Thus, the critical barrier to wellness is repetition—sticking to a new activity long enough for it to become integrated into daily practices. The repetition step is what trips most of us up. And the reason is simple: Inertia is a powerful force—a phenomenon that applies to humans as much as to Isaac Newton's apples.Because we are biologically programmed to conserve energy, we easily fall back on old habits, even if they don't serve our ultimate goals.

We need willpower as the force to overcome inertia. But repeatedly relying on willpower for wellness activities depletes our limited supply, leading us to eventually give up and revert to bad habits. One of the best studies on this topic comes from Katy Milkman, a Wharton colleague of mine, who looked at handwashing in hospitals, an important "wellness" behavior that can reduce patient infections and even deaths. Milkman and her colleagues followed over 4,000 health care workers at nearly three dozen hospitals who collectively had 13 million handwashing opportunities. They found that handwashing compliance consistently declined from the beginning to the end of a 12-hour work shift. Workers who engaged in more cognitively taxing activities—such as those with more patient responsibilities—demonstrated a greater decline in handwashing compliance. Time away from work—mental and physical recuperation—was associated with improvement in handwashing. Compliance did not bounce back overnight, but returned to baseline over several days. This indicates that cognitive fatigue can have a long-term impact on our ability to adopt wellness behaviors.

Another set of experiments by French researchers demonstrated how repetitive cognitive burden leads to worse decision-making and a tendency toward immediate gratification. Participants were asked to categorize a letter by type (vowel or consonant) or case (uppercase or lowercase), depending on the color. Adding to the mental challenge, the colors were frequently switched. At the end of the activity, the participants were asked to make a choice between getting $87 now or $100 later—immediate or delayed gratification. The participants' willpower diminished as they engaged in the cognitively challenging activity, and they increasingly gravitated toward more immediate rewards. MRI scans showed decreased activity in the area of the brain that controls complex executive functions like decision-making, planning, and weighing the outcomes of different choices. As the researchers conclude: "prior exertion of self-control [impairs] the ability to perform subsequent unrelated tasks that also require self-control." In other words, willpower can be fatigued and prevent the self-control necessary for adopting wellness behaviors.

These studies help us understand not only how to effectively harness willpower for wellness, but more importantly how to transition away from relying on willpower in order to adopt wellness behaviors. The first take-home message is to stay away from any wellness program that requires extreme and simultaneous changes in your diet, workouts, water intake, and reading. This is bound to fail. It will deplete your willpower, and fast. Instead, be like Benjamin Franklin, an expert in self-improvement who described his own practice of trying to adopt new habits in his *Autobiography*: "I judg'd it would be well not to distract my attention by attempting the whole at once." Focus on one change at a time. Commit to stop drinking sugary beverages, say, but don't simultaneously try to change your social media habits and take up running.

How do you establish a new routine?

There are four strategic steps that help to ensure the transition from initiation to repetition to routine practice of a wellness behavior. The first is to plan. Set a specific goal to start on a specific date at a specific time and place. Pick a date you will quit snacking or start going to the gym or not look at your phone in the hour before going to bed. Avoid vague declarations—delineate a specific plan and maybe write it down to commit yourself.

Second, identify triggers that might make you give up the new action, and plan what you will do when confronted by them. Maybe you are like Queen Victoria, who was prone to get hungry and faint at 3:30 p.m. Like her, you have your afternoon teatime with cookies. What about changing your teatime routine by munching on an apple and a handful of nuts? Or consider going for a short walk to get fresh air and touch base with a sibling instead of wandering into the kitchen past those oh-so-tempting cookies.

Third, have social supports. Adopting a wellness initiative with others to support and encourage you incentivizes maintaining the behavior. When I worked at the National Institutes of Health in Bethesda, Maryland, a friend and I would go out for a 4- or 5-mile run through Rock Creek Park two or three afternoons a week. We would talk through issues at work or at home, discuss research projects we were working on, or air whatever grievances were on our minds.

These runs were wellness grand slams, combining exercise, time with nature, and good social relations. It also didn't hurt that he was a psychiatrist and knew how to ask open-ended questions. Consequently, I always turned out to be the breathless one. That routine held for over a decade, until my colleague moved away, but running had become so integral to my well-being that I continued to run during work twice a week.

So, consider adopting a fitness or afternoon "snack" routine
with a friend. The expectation of having to show up to be with
a friend will help you—and them!—establish a lasting habit.

Finally, reward yourself with a job well done. Wellness
should not feel like a long series of deprivations. Positive feed-
back along the wellness path helps all of us keep going. For
most people, having immediate rewards is the best reinforce-
ment. Sometimes the rewards are directly from the activity—
enjoying the endorphins of exercise. Other times, we can
create incentives.

Katy Milkman developed what she calls "temptation bun-
dling" that combines "want activities"—listening to a popular
audiobook—with a wellness behavior—exercising at the gym.
The important trick was that the participants could *only* listen to the audiobooks while at the gym. Unsurprisingly, this
combination of a reward with a wellness behavior increased
gym attendance.

How many repetitions over how many days does it take to
form a new wellness habit? Expert views on this topic are all
over the place. Some lore has habit formation at 21 days. Others claim 66 days. Still others reference a range with an upper
limit of 254 days. (James Clear, of *Atomic Habits* fame, sum-
marizes the history of this variation.) Such variation tells you
that there is no precise answer and that habit formation is
contextual. It will vary by the type of behavior you are trying
to adopt, the magnitude of the change, the surrounding environmental cues, your social supports, and who you are.

One Canadian study offers some useful insight. Just after
New Year's, researchers followed people who newly joined
a gym to examine their formation of an exercise habit. The
participants reported their daily exercise patterns. People
who went less than 4 times a week were unlikely to exercise

at 12 weeks, but those who exercised 4 or more times a week for the first 6 weeks developed a habit that endured for 12 weeks or more. As the researchers put it, "consistency [that is, repetition] was the most important predictor followed by low behavioral complexity." The takeaway: Keep the routines simple and repeat them at least 4 times a week and in about 6 weeks you'll seem to have a habit.

Keep in mind that even small changes can make a huge difference—as long as those changes are strategic. But they can't be too small. Micro or tiny changes, like writing down one thing you're grateful for every day, are just not sufficient for wellness and improving your health. The science of motivation has shown that seeing results is an effective motivator to keep going. Even brief, low-impact physical activity, like 20 minutes of yoga first thing in the morning or in the evening before dinner, makes a measurable difference. And building on your progress increases the returns. Starting with 20 minutes of walking three days a week can progress to a light jog and then ultimately a run over a series of months.

The same goes for nutrition: The most important action is to wean yourself off eating foods that promote disease and focus on a few relatively minor dietary changes. Even small changes can have a major impact. For example, a recent study found that daily consumption of at least 7 grams of olive oil a day, just over a teaspoon and a half, was associated with a 28% decrease in dementia-related death. Dementia is the greatest fear of many Americans, and this study suggests that you can reduce your risk by simply switching from store-bought salad dressing to homemade dressing with olive oil. And don't forget to reward yourself! Have that scoop of ice cream when you accomplish a change. That might not be in your diet, but it is nothing to avoid or to apologize for either.

———

When I began brainstorming for this book, a friend guilt-ily took me aside and confessed, "I know I shouldn't drink diet sodas. I've tried to stop, but I just can't." She looked at me as if she had just drowned a puppy and was prepared to be severely chastised.

But my response was anything but a rebuke. "I know how you feel. But remember, I'm a professor. 90% is an A. Even a B is a good grade. The same goes for wellness. You don't have to get 100% to live a long, healthy life."

I'll readily admit my own "failings" on the wellness front. I love to bake desserts. One of my favorites is my mother's cheesecake recipe. Three packages of full-fat cream cheese, plus 1 cup of sugar, and plenty of butter in the crust—all that goodness goes right to the coronary arteries like a heat-seeking missile. A slice of cheesecake is not listed on any known wellness diet.

But I don't sneak pieces when no one is looking. Indeed, I am proud to serve it to my friends at dinner parties—or my brother on his birthday—because I think it is the best cheese-cake there is. Even a long life is too short to feel guilty or ashamed for not being perfect. Or to miss out completely on the things you love.

Wellness and longevity are not like taxes or an Olympic gymnastics routine, where a little mistake can mean a fine from the IRS or losing a medal. Wellness is about the over-all course of a life—your lifestyle—not each particular action. Benjamin Franklin was never able to achieve his goal of order-liness. His life was always a bit of a mess. But he was still a towering genius who lived productively and mentally engaged to the age of 84. And my friend's diet sodas may not promote wellness, but combined with other behaviors—like sharing dinner with friends—they won't cost her 10 days or even 10 seconds in the longevity sweepstakes. Indeed, trying to do every single wellness rule every single day will exhaust your willpower and lead to frustration and failure. Wellness ought to be in the background: an unconscious part of your lifestyle, not an obsession.

And even scrupulously adhering to the six wellness behaviors outlined in this book will not guarantee a long, happy life. Unexpected good and bad, things happen that we cannot control. So don't sweat the occasional lapse. But incorporating these tweaks into your daily routine can dramatically improve your odds at long-term good health without allowing them to consume you.

As the eminent British rabbi Jonathan Sacks once wrote: "We defeat death, not by living forever but by living by values that live forever." Wellness is the way to love and nourish our family and friends, perform good deeds of loving kindness, enrich our communities, and leave the world a better place. That's why this book holds two truths at once: Longevity and wellness aren't everything, and yet a long and healthy life creates more space to pursue all we love and believe to be important. Those are the things that matter.

1

Don't Be a Schmuck

Avoiding Self-Destructive Risks

As a 16-year-old growing up in the northern suburbs of Chicago, I hated relying on my mom for rides. I desperately wanted a car. Equipped with $500 of the bar mitzvah money I saved, every week I scoured classified ads in the city's free newspaper—*The Reader*—for cars that might fall within my budget. My heart was set on a Volvo or a Saab. They were likely to be stick shift, and in my teenager's imagination, they seemed cool.

Occasionally, my dad would catch me poring over the paper and say, "Don't be a schmuck! You don't need a car, and you can't afford one either." Undeterred, I kept searching and finally, finally, about 7 months after I got my license, I found it ... my dream car. For $400, a green stick shift Volvo 122 with four doors. My brother Ari and I took my bar mitzvah money out of the bank and got a ride down to the seller's home. When we pulled up, we were glad to see that the car looked as described in the ad. More excited by the minute, I walked around the car to check for dents in the body or scratches in

the paint. I confirmed that the interior was well maintained
and that all the windows worked. I slid into the driver's seat
to take it for a test run. The car drove well: The clutch worked
smoothly, and the transmission shifted easily from first to
second to third (we could not go fast enough to get into fourth
gear on Chicago side streets). After some negotiation, we got
the beautiful old Volvo for $300. Driving the new car home, we
were elated and felt accomplished. We got what we wanted—
and at a bargain that would really appeal to my financially
frugal (aka cheapskate) father.

As we proudly pulled into the driveway, my father walked
out of the side door of our house and asked what we were
doing. I remember confidently telling him, "It's almost an
antique, but it drives well!" His response: "What schmucks!"
He ordered us to back out of the driveway so he could pull out
his car. That was the eureka moment. The car would not go
into reverse.

My brother and I had thought we were discerning, focused
on doing our due diligence before driving away with that car.
But in retrospect, we were so distracted by the amazing possibility of owning our dream car that we had turned a blind
eye to the essentials. We were schmucks. I still haven't lived
this down. To this day, whenever my family thinks I am being
stupid or they want to niggle me for something, they chide me
with "It's almost an antique!"

I've learned that my Dad's saying holds true for wellness,
health, and longevity. Just as it is easy to get distracted by a
car's polished, shiny exterior before ensuring its basic functionality, it's easy to get lost in the flood of wellness tips, diet
fads, and exercise recommendations while overlooking the
first true rule of a life well lived: *Don't be a schmuck.*

Everything we do in life has risks. If you go skiing, you

might break a leg—or worse, smash your head on a tree and end up with a concussion. If you try an adventurous new food, you might discover an allergy. But you don't need—and shouldn't seek—to eliminate all activities with risk to avoid being a schmuck. You don't need to pack yourself in bubble wrap. Just avoid the things that carry a high risk of serious irreversible harm—dying, damaging your brain, becoming paralyzed, or losing the ability to live consciously and deliberately—without taking extra precautions. For instance, I ride a Vespa-like electric scooter. As scootering becomes more common, accidents are increasing. But the risk of really serious accidents involving traumatic brain injury can be reduced—although not eliminated—by wearing a helmet and not scootering in dangerous road conditions, such as at night or in rain or snow. Risk can also be minimized by not driving recklessly—like driving through red lights or the wrong way down a one-way street. This risk reduction exercise extends beyond scootering to the many aspects of day-to-day life that inherently involve risk. However, millions of Americans still regularly make choices that dramatically increase the risk of serious, irreversible harm.

When it comes to self-destructive risks, there are eight major opportunities to make high-impact choices to avoid the most common and serious threats to your life. Like much of wellness, *not* doing stupid things may be the most important action you can take. My aim in this chapter is to make explicit some of the most common "schmuck moves" and further the evidence-based case for avoiding them. Ensuring you do the boring things—like brushing your teeth twice a day—is the best way to begin your journey to wellness and longevity. Before following any new-fangled advice, which rarely has supporting data and won't add much to the length or quality of your life, make sure you aren't shooting yourself in the foot, literally or figuratively.

Hands down, the first schmuck move is **smoking**, and the

right thing to do is to quit. I *would* tell you not to start smoking, but anyone reading this book is likely to already be over 18, and virtually no one starts smoking once they're old enough to vote. It is primarily teenagers, whose prefrontal cortex is not fully developed, who succumb to the slick advertising from Big Tobacco. Worse yet, these ads are targeted at minority, low-income, and poorly educated individuals, and their effect is amplified by a culture that places enormous social pressure on teens to smoke. Indeed, the habit is so nasty that over 70% of current smokers want to quit. So, the first smart move is to ensure that any teenager or young adult you know doesn't start—and then, for anyone who does smoke, to quit.

Why? Because, on average, a smoker loses 10 years of life compared with a nonsmoker, and a heavy smoker loses 13 years. Each cigarette a smoker lights up shortens their life by approximately 20 minutes. Whether through heart disease, cancer, stroke, emphysema, or dozens of other conditions, there may be no other human behavior that so drastically and clearly reduces health and longevity. And it's never too late to quit—the health benefits of quitting at any age are equally clear. Quitting by age 44, for example, will add 9 years back to your life expectancy. In 2024, researchers in South Korea published a study looking at over 5 million people and found that those who had smoked a pack a day for 8 years or less and then quit had no higher risk of cardiovascular disease compared with never-smokers. Quitting cigarettes before the damage becomes irreversible is definitely a wellness move.

Now, smoking is addictive, and quitting is incredibly hard. My own mom—a woman I personally know to possess incredible strength—has never been able to permanently quit. And if you're questioning her determination or fortitude, just remember that she raised me and my brothers: I can assure you that requires one tough lady. But even with the help of her sons, who used sewing needles to poke holes in her cigarettes, the habit held fast. Consequently, I have a lot of empathy for people who have struggled to quit smoking.

The addictive nature of tobacco products means that very few people can do it cold turkey. The most famous cold turkey case I know of is President Dwight Eisenhower. He was a four-pack-a-day chain smoker, especially during World War II, when he was supreme commander organizing the D-Day invasion. One day in 1949, after his physician urged him to cut back to one pack, he just quit. Like many people trying to stop a bad habit, Ike found quitting a lot easier than weaning himself. But Ike had this crazy habit of stuffing his pockets with cigarettes and giving them to smokers. Why? According to then mayor of Detroit Jerome Cavanaugh:

> The President told me that he used to go around with cigarettes in all his pockets while he was trying to give up smoking. He would pass them out to other smokers but not touch them himself, because this gave him a feeling of accomplishment and superiority.

Ike never smoked for the rest of his life. Despite decades of smoking, having quit when he was in his late 50s, he lived to be 78 years old at a time when the life expectancy of an American male was just 67 years.

Who knows how people who just stop do it. It might be a sense of clarity about the tremendous costs in terms of lost days and years from smoking. It might also be part of a change in lifestyle brought on by a significant event, like a marriage, birth, or trauma. Even if you're not like Ike, you can still stop smoking. But remember, it may take multiple attempts to actually stop. In fact, it has long been thought that it takes, on average, somewhere between 5 and 14 attempts before some-

one succeeds in quitting. More recently, Canadian researchers found that the number is more likely to be 30 or more
attempts. This means you shouldn't stop trying even after a
failed attempt or two. Use the decades of good research revealing what behaviors actually help people quit.

One proven strategy involves the following steps. First,
plan. Set a date to quit, and don't keep postponing it. Second,
identify and write down the contexts or environmental triggers that ignite your cravings for a cigarette, such as drinking in a bar or going out to a party or going to a coffee shop
with another friend who smokes. Then avoid these trigger-
ing situations to the extent possible; if you can't fully avoid
them, reduce them and plan how you will respond to cravings and whatever triggers your desire to smoke. Third, start
using nicotine replacement therapy—a patch, gum, lozenges,
or nasal spray—and/or non-nicotine drugs like bupropion
and varenicline. When you get a craving, give your mouth
something else to do, like chewing gum—xylitol gum to avoid
cavities—or sucking candy. Mix in other wellness activities
that help and distract from the craving—exercise and sleep
help. But maybe the most important thing is to have support,
or as the National Center for Health Research puts it, "call
in reinforcements." Have family, friends, or a support group
to encourage and talk with you, especially when you are having cravings. You even might want to quit with a friend, so
you can help each other when the going gets especially tough.
Finally, reach out to organizations like the American Lung
Association or the American Cancer Society for free support
to help quit.

Quitting smoking is hard. An addiction to cigarettes is both
biological and psychological. Not succeeding the first time
doesn't make you a failure. It just means addiction is a hard
thing to tackle. Struggling with an addiction doesn't make you

a schmuck—but giving up does. That extra decade of life you will gain back is surely worth it.

Lots of people think vaping is the best way to wean yourself off cigarettes. This is controversial. E-cigarettes were initially dreamed up as a mechanism to help people quit smoking. A recent analysis of 90 research trials of vaping done by British researchers for the Cochrane collaborative concluded that vaping was better than other forms of nicotine replacement and non-nicotine treatments in getting smokers to quit. Vaping likely enabled an "additional four quitters per 100 smokers." Hence, the British government supports vaping for quitting and has "provided 1 million smokers in England a vape to help them quit smoking."

However, the FDA has not approved e-cigarettes as a smoking cessation device in the United States. And after reviewing the data, the United States Preventive Services Task Force (USPSTF) also does not recommend vaping to quit smoking. There are several good reasons why leading US health agencies have not endorsed vaping for smoking cessation.

First, in the real world—outside of controlled clinical trials—it appears that vaping is additive to cigarette smoking and does not help people quit. For instance, researchers at the University of California, San Diego enrolled nearly 46,000 adults in a study and interviewed them over the next 4 years. About a quarter of the daily smokers used e-cigarettes. Just under 10% had quit over the next year. Surprisingly, that was the same percentage of smokers who had quit without using e-cigarettes. And the study was repeated with newer data but with the same result: "No evidence that cessation rates [among smokers using e-cigarettes] differed from closely matched smokers who did not use e-cigarettes." Even worse, a subsequent study of vaping showed that smokers who are trying to quit and simultaneously vaped actually smoked longer than those who did not vape. In the technical language of researchers, "vaping was not associated with increased smoking cessation and was associated with reduced tobacco abstinence." That double negative—reduced abstinence—really means that people who vaped daily smoked more, about 15% longer. As the USPSTF put it, "the balance of benefits and harms (of vaping) cannot be determined." Trading one schmuck move for another is still schmucky.

So what is the scale of the vaping problem in the United States? Vaping hit a boom in the mid 2010s, before the US surgeon general declared it an epidemic among America's youth in 2018. The next year, youth vaping peaked, when nearly 30% of high schoolers and over 10% of middle schoolers reported vaping at least once during the previous month. That is over 5 million middle and high schoolers vaping. Luckily, the federal and state crackdown brought the number of kids vaping way down to just over 1.6 million in 2024. But that's still 1.6 million too many.

The story for adults is more appalling. According to the Centers for Disease Control and Prevention (CDC), "Between 2019 and 2023, the percentage of adults who used electronic cigarettes increased significantly for all age groups, except those ages 18–20 and 65 and older." These figures demonstrate the increasing popularity of vaping by those who can purchase vapes legally.

This leads to the second point. Through various marketing ploys, vaping has become not only its own deleterious beast, but also a gateway to cigarettes for those who otherwise might never have smoked a cigarette. A 2017 review of over 17,000 adolescents and young adults found that e-cigarette use was associated with greater risk for subsequent cigarette smoking initiation. Vaping does not deter smoking but rather normalizes smoking—which portends poorly for keeping people from ever trying cigarettes.

Third, while vaping may be safer than smoking today, that doesn't make it safe. Indeed, e-cigarettes have health problems of their own. Vaping is just another way to inhale nicotine or THC (the primary psychoactive compound in weed). Accompanying each inhalation are thousands of chemicals. Not all the chemicals in vaping smoke are known, but some of the known ones are terrible for you, causing lung and heart disease. Michael Blaha, director of clinical research at the John Hopkins Ciccarone Center for the Prevention of Cardiovascular Disease, recenty concluded a nearly four-year study with over 250,000 people who either (1) exclusively smoked cigarettes, (2) exclusively vaped, (3) smoked cigarettes and vaped, or (4) neither smoked cigarettes nor vaped ever. After about 4 years, the cigarette smokers had significantly increased their risks for hypertension, type 2 diabetes, emphysema, heart failure, and atherosclerotic cardiovascular disease. No surprise there. Interestingly, the researchers found that exclusively vaping was not significantly associated with type 2 diabetes or cardiovascular disease, but it was significantly associated with emphysema. As Blaha succinctly summarized it, "e-cigarettes have definite potential health risks, although the risks may be less than what is seen for traditional combustible cigarette smoking alone." Emphasizing this point, back in 2024, Australia passed a law to impose barriers to buying e-cigarettes, including limiting the sale of vaping products to pharmacies and requiring consultation with a pharmacist before purchase.

Not only does vaping expose kids to lung damage, but even worse, it dulls their brains. A recent study showed that college students who vaped scored lower on tests of learning, memory, problem solving and critical thinking. Not surprisingly, there was a dose response: The more that young people vaped, the worse their scores. And like cigarettes, the nicotine in vaping can lead to dysregulation in brain activity related to attention, impulse control, and mood.

Finally, the long-term health risks of vaping are unknown. Unlike with cigarettes, we don't yet have decades of data about how much time each vape puff takes off your life. After all, lifelong vape users are still mostly young adults. So even if vaping aids with cigarette smoking cessation or can be called safer than cigarettes today, to take up vaping today merely swaps a known harm for an unknown one.

Not being a schmuck means educating young people in your life to prevent them from being played for fools by this new generation of tobacco companies pitching vaping as the cooler, healthier alternative. The science is clear: The best way to not be a schmuck is to not start smoking or vaping.

Cigarettes and vapes are schmuck moves; for many people so is weed, especially chronic use. Recreational weed is now legal in 24 US states and the District of Columbia. It is also legal or decriminalized in Canada, Germany, Luxembourg, Malta, Mexico, and a few other countries. Many other countries allow it for medical use. Consequently, use has increased in all demographics—all age-groups, men and women, and, surprisingly, even among pregnant women. The highest use is in the 18–25 age-group, but even among Americans over 50, as many as 21% used cannabis at least once in the last year.

Today weed has about 3 times more THC, the active ingredient, than was in the marijuana of old. This means its effects on the brain are much more potent.

The short-term effects of weed are well known and not really different from alcohol use. Feeling relaxed, happy, and calm—that is why people use weed. And for some, especially cancer patients, weed can counter nausea and offer pain relief.

However, there are immediate short-term coordination problems and slower reaction times, especially important for driving and athletic performance. Since legalization, some studies estimate that annual deaths from traffic accidents increased by about 1,400 due to cannabis use among drivers.

But what makes weed a schmuck move is chronic use that has three bad effects. The first is addiction. In the 1960s, it was claimed that pot was not addictive. But today it is estimated that 10% of pot users will become addicted, and the rate is higher (about 17%) if the users start before age 18.

More worrisome is weed use among pregnant women. Surveys show that about 1 in 16 pregnant women admit to having used weed in the previous 30 days, but urine sampling suggests that about half of pregnant women who use weed deny using it. So it may be that 1 in 10 pregnant women or more are using weed. And weed use during pregnancy is associated with worse outcomes for both the mother and the newborn baby. For moms there is increased risk of gaining too much weight—those munchies—hypertension and preeclampsia, as well as detachment of the placenta from the uterus, which compromises the baby's oxygen supply. For babies cannabis use by moms is associated with lower birth weight, popping out preterm, brain development problems, including long-term problems, and increased rate of ending up in the neonatal intensive care unit.

Finally, for all people, chronic use over years is bad for the brain. Tests of working memory and executive functions—retaining and using information as well as decision-making, problem-solving, and motor skills—show that about two-thirds of long-term cannabis users had reduced brain activity. A 45-year study in New Zealand enrolled over 1,000 people born in 1972–73 and followed them until age 45. Cannabis use was assessed 6 times between ages 18 and 45, and IQ tests and other brain tests were administered multiple times. As the authors write:

> Long-term cannabis users showed IQ decline from childhood to midlife (mean = -5.5 IQ points), poorer learning and processing speed relative to their childhood IQ, and informant-reported memory and attention problems. These deficits were specific to long-term cannabis users because they were either not present or were smaller among long-term tobacco users, long-term alcohol users, midlife recreational cannabis users, and cannabis quitters.

Chronic weed makes people slower, less able to focus and remember things. Indeed, the results indicate that chronic cannabis use is like early cognitive impairment. Occasional recreational use of weed is probably okay, but chronic use and use during pregnancy seem like schmuck moves. So try to reduce or even quit by decreasing the potency of your weed and how frequently you use it. And use the same steps that cigarette smokers use to quit.

Next on the schmuck list is **alcohol**. Heavy drinking (15 drinks or more a week for men and 8 or more for women), binge drinking (5 drinks or more per occasion for men and 4 or more for women), and drinking alone are incontrovertibly bad for you. The lingering controversy is really just about light alcohol consumption for adults over 40.

Worldwide, the use of alcohol is "the 10th most relevant risk factor (for death), responsible for over 1.8 million deaths from various alcohol-attributable causes." In 2020, alcohol was the leading risk factor for death for men aged 15 to 48 years. A 2018 *Lancet* systematic review found even infrequent consumption carried risk and concluded that "the safest level of drinking is none."

Yet, in 2022, a different publication from *The Lancet* by

researchers from the Institute for Health Metrics and Evaluation stated that for people over age 40, drinking up to about 1.5 standard drinks a day may provide some health benefits—namely, reduced risk of cardiovascular disease, stroke, and diabetes. They reported, however, that there are no health benefits to drinking alcohol, only health risks, for people under age 40.

Other studies support the possibility of health benefits with moderation. For instance, a British study of over 135,000 people published in 2024 found that light drinking during meals and drinking wine generally showed some slight benefit for people with health-related risk factors and who lived in deprived areas. Another study with over 50,000 participants showed that light to moderate drinking—between 1 and 14 drinks per week—is associated with a reduction in stroke or heart attack. The positive impact is a lot stronger for men than for women. Also, this heart benefit was most noticeable in people with heart disease.

However, in 2023, the World Health Organization (WHO) pointed out, "There are no studies that would demonstrate that the potential beneficial effects of light and moderate drinking on cardiovascular diseases and type 2 diabetes outweigh the cancer risk associated with these same levels of alcohol consumption for individual consumers." After all, alcohol is causally linked to seven different types of cancer. Ultimately, both WHO and the United Kingdom's chief medical officer have declared that there is "no safe level of alcohol consumption."

So why don't I advise everyone to give up booze altogether? As I have learned working in public health, in my clinical work with patients, and even in my conversations within my own family, people tune out recommendations that are too extreme. They shop for an opinion they like better—and the

Internet makes that all too easy. And since research from rigorous academic journals offers conflicting takeaways, there is no clear answer.

Whether they verbalize it or not, people seem to think that human beings have been drinking since the dawn of time. Moreover, plenty of cases seem to support some level of alcohol consumption. All those people in the Blue Zones who regularly live healthy lives into their 90s routinely tipple a little with meals. How bad can drinking be if it has existed forever and is a habit of some of the healthiest, longest-lived people on earth?

The behavior and routines of people in Blue Zones remind us that it's important to consider *how* people drink alcohol. As we will see, regularly socializing with friends has a huge positive impact on health and well-being. So, while research suggests having a drink a day may be neutral or increase your risk of death, that is probably outweighed by the benefits of time with friends. The upshot is that drinking alone is always a bad idea, but an occasional social drink is not against the doctor's orders.

If you do choose to drink—in the company of friends and family—make sure you have a plan for how to safely get home. Remember that drinking and driving don't mix. Even small amounts of alcohol impair judgment, coordination, and reaction time. It is shocking how frequently people drink and drive and how little alcohol it takes to compromise your driving.

Every month, 1.2% of adults drive "after having too much to drink." Further, the CDC's data show that the number of self-reported drunk driving incidents among adults has been well over 100 million every year since 1993. At the federal blood alcohol limit—0.08%—a person is 300% more likely to have a car accident. Indeed, even for blood alcohol levels that are significantly lower than the federal standard—at 0.05%—a driver is still pretty impaired, with a 38% higher risk of an accident than a nondrinker. This is one reason that the blood alcohol limits in much of Europe are lower than in the United States. Though incredibly risky, drunk driving is also incredibly common. Every 39 minutes an American dies in a drunk driving accident—over 13,000 per year. If you drink, use a rideshare service—they are associated with a reduction in driving-related trauma, fatalities, and DUI convictions. Don't be a schmuck—don't drink and drive.

Drinking isn't the only way to drive like a schmuck. Texting while driving increases the risk of a crash 23-fold. When you take your eyes and mind off the road, you can't react quickly to anything that happens. Distracted drivers tend to swerve into other lanes. They don't react when a green light turns red or a red light turns green. In 2010 the National Safety Council estimated that 1.6 million accidents are caused by cell phone distraction. In 2019, nearly 425,000 people were injured and more than 3,000 were killed in crashes involving a distracted driver. All driving deaths dropped from a peak of 56,278 in 1972 to a 50-year low of 35,303 in 2011, but then began increasing again in 2014. Precisely *why* is debated, but the addiction to smart phones and texting is a leading culprit. One potential clue: The iPhone was first sold in 2007 and became ubiquitous in 2010. And remember, it's not only *your* life that's at risk. So don't be a schmuck. Don't text and drive. Put that phone out of arm's reach when you're behind the wheel.

The Beatles famously sang "Here comes the sun," appealing to the fact that we all love to catch some rays. My brothers and I spent—or maybe misspent—many summers hours of our youth hanging out on beaches, swimming and body surfing. And we weren't religious about the sunscreen. And little boys in Chicago are hardly unique. Think of those few sunny winter days in Sweden when older ladies bundle up to sit on park benches, tilting their faces to get some sun.

Sunshine warms us, invigorates us, and lifts our mood. Indeed, the sun's rays stimulate the production and release of serotonin, a brain hormone associated with good feelings and a sense of joy. Furthermore, decreased exposure to sunlight in the winter, and the subsequent decreased levels of serotonin, causes seasonal affective disorder, or SAD.

But the benefits of sunlight don't mean you should skip your sunscreen routine. We all need at least 10 to 30 minutes of natural sunlight every day, especially in the morning. The sun streaming through our eyes regulates our circadian rhythm and improves our mood. Sunlight on our skin is necessary to convert cholesterol into vitamin D, which is associated with strong bones, a healthy immune system, cardiovascular health, and good muscle function. Too much sunlight, though, can cause deadly melanomas and can prematurely wrinkle our skin. The solution is clothing and sunscreen. Randomized and population studies in Australia, Norway, and other countries show that clothing and sunscreen (SPF over 30) reduces the melanoma risk by 50%—particularly among children and young people.

Misinformation on TikTok and other social media channels has many people—especially young people—taking dangerous risks with sun exposure. A recent survey by the American Academy of Dermatology showed that "52% of Gen Z adults were unaware of one or more sunburn risks, such as increased risk of developing skin cancer or premature skin aging." Even worse, 28% of them said that "getting a tan was more important to them than preventing skin cancer." Another survey by a cancer institute revealed that 14% of adults under 35 believe that wearing sunscreen is more dangerous than direct sun exposure. These shocking beliefs will likely be reflected in rising rates of melanoma.

Some of the concerns seem to stem from studies demonstrating that oxybenzone, a common sunscreen ingredient, can disrupt endocrine function and cause other health problems when fed to rats in high doses You are not a rat. You don't eat sunscreen. And you would have to use sunscreen for nearly 200 years to get the same amount of oxybenzone exposure as the rats in the experiment. Still worried? You can easily avoid sunscreens with oxybenzone and use those with the mineral sunblocks zinc oxide, titanium dioxide, or other safe ingredients. Protecting your skin from excessive cancer-causing ultraviolet (UV) rays is one of the easiest and most effective health choices you can make. And dying of melanoma is one of the most horrible ways to go because it has the capacity to metastasize all over the body—from the brain to the lungs to the bones—causing excruciating symptoms and mental confusion.

Tanning salons are also a schmuck move. I understand the appeal of having a tanned body, but tanning beds fry you with UVA, ultraviolet light that goes deep into your skin and damages your cells' DNA. A 2007 review found that exposure to sunbeds before age 35 increases the risk of melanoma by 75%. A more recent review and meta-analysis from 2021 found that "using tanning beds before age 20 can increase your chances of developing melanoma by 47%, and the risk increases with each use." And did I mention that UVA accelerates wrinkles? Moreover, tanning salons don't offer the kind of UVB light that produces vitamin D. There are no physical health benefits from tanning beds whatsoever—only risks.

Indeed, I am proud to have been part of the team that suc-

ceeded in adding a 10% tax on indoor tanning services in the
Affordable Care Act (ACA) to discourage this behavior.

Don't listen to schmucks spreading false ideas and misinformation about **vaccines**. Take your shots. Vaccines remove
risk and worry from your life. They are worth the momen-
tary pain for living with much lower risk of many cancers,
paralysis, painful shingles, pneumonia, or brain damage. Your
grandparents worried that their children might contract polio
and end up in an iron lung or wheelchair or dead. No parent
has to worry about that today because of vaccines.

Vaccines have allowed us to eliminate smallpox, one of the
real scourges of history that has killed over 300 million people
worldwide since 1900 alone. Polio is also on the verge of being
eliminated by vaccines. Many other diseases, including measles, rubella, diphtheria, and haemophilus influenzae (Hib),
also experienced a 99%+ decrease in prevalence between
1900 and 2016 because of vaccines. Just look at Table 1 for a
glimpse of all the diseases we have vaccines for and how few
people die each year from those diseases in the United States.

These diseases used to infect millions and kill thousands
of people each year, and they were particularly dangerous for
vulnerable populations like infants and immunosuppressed
people. If you stub your toe on a rusty nail, you don't have to
worry about dying of tetanus anymore. We live in a country
without deadly epidemics of whooping cough. And we used to
live in a country without deadly measles outbreaks. Measles
was officially eliminated from the United States in 2000. But
then anti-vaxxer parents decided not to vaccinate their children, producing multiple serious outbreaks. In 2025, there
has been an especially bad outbreak in West Texas and New
Mexico, with a near 20% rate of hospitalizations and 3 deaths
and counting. The child who died in Texas was unvaccinated,

and her death was the first in the United States from measles in a decade.

Table 1: Deaths from Vaccine Preventable Diseases

Disease for Which We Have a Vaccine	How Many Die from the Disease in the US
PERTUSSIS (WHOOPING COUGH)	10 deaths in 2024 (total of 9 deaths in the prior 3 years, 2021–2023)
DIPHTHERIA	0 deaths a year (last recorded case in 1997)
MEASLES	3 deaths between Jan 2024 and June 2025 (the first deaths since 2015 and all were unvaccinated)
RABIES	Less than 10 deaths a year
TETANUS	Average of 2 deaths a year since 2000
CHICKENPOX	Less than 30 deaths a year
HEPATITIS B	Less than 2,000 deaths a year
MENINGOCOCCUS	Less than 50 deaths a year (total of 93 deaths in 3 years between 2020 and 2022)
RUBELLA	No deaths per year
HAEMOPHILUS INFLUENZAE (HIB)	No higher than background rate of infant deaths from SIDS and other conditions

There is one other vaccine that is becoming even more important to take: the shingles vaccine, Shingrix. Data indicate that people who get this vaccine have the added benefit of a lower risk of developing dementia. Since the vaccine effectively prevents painful shingles and may reduce chances of dementia . . . what's not to like?

To maintain this safer, healthier way of life, we have to keep getting our vaccines. You might have heard stories of people harmed by a vaccine and suspect that anti-vaxxers may be onto something. As with any medication or drug, there are rare instances of side effects and unexpected outcomes. But the risks of all approved vaccines are exceedingly low, especially compared with the things you do every day like driving your car—even without drinking or texting. The lifetime risk of dying in a car crash is 1 in 95. The lifetime risk of dying from a vaccine is . . . well, it is so low it is hard to calculate. And the talk about deaths from the COVID-19 vaccines is just plain wrong. By mid-July of 2021—about 7 months into COVID-19 vaccinations—about 340 million doses of the COVID-19 vaccine had been administered to Americans. At that time, the highest estimate was that the vaccine *might* have been associated with 6,207 deaths—a rate of 0.0018% per dose. But by the end of July 2021, there were 610,000 COVID-related deaths in the United States. Furthermore, in Washington state, the rate of being hospitalized or dying from COVID-19 was more than 3 times higher for unvaccinated adults between the ages 35 and 64 compared with COVID-19 vaccinated adults. And among unvaccinated seniors in Washington state, the rate of dying from COVID-19 was 1.8 times higher than for those vaccinated. Another meta-analysis published in 2023 on over 21 million people found that unvaccinated patients were nearly 2.5 times more likely to die from COVID-19 than vaccinated patients. What's the bigger threat—the vaccine or being unvaccinated and getting infected with COVID-19?

It is understandable to point out the deeply unfortunate person who suffers an adverse event from a vaccine. But since 1974, over 150 million lives have been saved by vaccination worldwide. It is much harder to "see" these millions who do *not* get polio or die from measles or whooping cough than those few individuals with adverse side effects. We cannot identify who would have gotten polio and lived a normal life but for the vaccine. There is no one to "see" because with vaccines, vaccinated people do not suffer from the disease.

While it's reasonable to weigh the risks and benefits, there's really no contest when it comes to approved vaccines. Overall, the risks of a severe reaction from a vaccine are exceedingly low. To provide a comparison, we can consider the safety of vaccines and peanut butter for children. For vaccines, life-threatening allergic reactions occur in approximately 1.3 out of every million doses. Meanwhile, out of the 2% of the kids who are allergic to peanuts, nearly 3% of them experience life-threatening allergic reactions every year. If you do the math, that's about 600 cases of life-threatening allergic reactions per million kids. If we assume the rate of 1.3 allergic reactions per million vaccine doses also applies to children, then peanut butter is more than 450 times more dangerous than vaccines are for all children.

Like vaccines, **cancer screening** is an important preventive medical intervention. Unfortunately, in recent years Americans have been avoiding cancer screening tests in increasingly larger numbers. For instance, according to the American Cancer Society, 1.1 million fewer women got breast cancer screening and 4.4 million fewer women got cervical cancer screening between 2019 and 2021. That drop was partially driven by the COVID-19 pandemic. However, the percentage of women aged 21 to 65 years up-to-date on cervical cancer screening has been falling since 2000. One survey in 2024 found that nearly 7 in 10 US adults were behind in at

least one routine cancer screening. That is after the pandemic
had ended. Undoubtedly there are excesses in routine health
testing in America—but avoiding mammograms, Pap smears,
and colonoscopies will only increase cancer-related deaths.
Colonoscopies, mammograms, and Pap smears save lives by
detecting cancers early. For instance, there is a lot of observational evidence that people who get screening colonoscopies
have a 40–69% lower chance of developing colorectal cancer
and about a 29–88% lower chance of dying from colorectal
cancer. Most of the US colorectal cancer deaths are attributable to missed screening opportunities. According to a 2022
landmark randomized-controlled trial of over 80,000 people
published in *The New England Journal of Medicine*, those who
got a colonoscopy saw about a 30% reduction in colon cancer risk and a 50% reduction in colon cancer death compared
with those who "went about their usual care, which did not
include regular colonoscopy screening." Given the reduction
in risk they provide, colonoscopies are well worth the bowel
preparation—which is, admittedly, pretty miserable. The good
news is that the prep only lasts a day. With the very worrisome uptick of colorectal cancer in people under 50, it is more
important than ever to get colonoscopies starting no later
than age 45.

If you are between 50 and 80 and you smoke or were a
smoker in the last 15 years, a low-dose CT scan to screen for
lung cancer is essential. Through early detection, these scans
can reduce the risk of dying from lung cancer by 20%. A bonus
is that it's free! (I am proud to have been a part of the ACA
team that ensured that these types of preventive tests are
available to Americans without deductibles or co-pays.)

For women, mammograms have simultaneously become de
rigueur, although slightly controversial. Let's start with what's
not controversial: All women should have mammograms every

other year between the ages of 45 and 74. There is no scientific debate around this point. However, the current controversy lies in whether to start screening earlier, at age 40, and whether mammograms lead to overdiagnosis and overtreatment of women with small tumors that would not cause serious harm, much less death, if left untreated. In April 2024, the US Preventive Services Task Force changed it guidelines to recommend starting at age 40. Breast cancer is much less common at this age but when discovered tends to be more advanced and aggressive.

The chance of a screening detecting breast cancer in a women aged 40 to 49 is about 1 in 750. Finding cancer in women aged 50 and over is about twice as likely. However, false positives, leading to more tests and potential biopsies, are common in younger women, occurring in 10–12% of mammograms for women between ages 40 and 49. I do not dismiss the uncertainty and anxiety generated by these false positives and understand why some women are therefore reluctant. So I believe whether to start mammograms at 40 or 45 is one of those judgment calls best left to a patient and her physician because the science is not definitive. But we do know for certain that all women born in the United States have a 13.1% lifetime chance of developing breast cancer. Regardless of when you start, it's a big mistake to forego mammogram screening and face that risk unprepared.

Women should also get Papanicolaou tests (Pap smears) and human papillomavirus (HPV) testing. Given the widespread availability of HPV vaccines and Pap smears, no woman should die of cervical cancer. But only 61% of teens are up-to-date on their HPV vaccine, and coverage began to stagnate in 2022. Further, nearly 25% of eligible women aren't getting their Pap smears, and the number of unscreened women has been going up, not down. The result is that over

4,000 American women (and 350,000 women worldwide) die, mostly unnecessarily, from cervical cancer each year. Get screened. Between the ages of 20 and 29, women should get a Pap smear every 3 years. Between 30 and 65, women should get a Pap smear combined with HPV testing every 5 years.

Getting screened is important, but stopping screening at the appropriate age is also important. Unless given a good reason by your doctor, I recommend that you *not* have Pap smears after 65 or colonoscopies or mammograms after age 75. And no low-dose CT scans after 80.

As the Joe Biden situation showed, the prostate-specific antigen (PSA) screening test for prostate cancer is much more complex and confusing. We should be clear about the guidelines and what is recommended. But let me be upfront—PSA is a bad test and I am against it. I think it is way overused.

Paradoxically, against my strong opinion and strong will, I have been tested four times. It's been forced on me.

The first time was when I was finished with having children and getting a vasectomy. As I was getting on the procedure table, the urologist said, "We're going to get some blood from you to test for prostate cancer."

"I don't want the PSA test. I am an oncologist and don't think the test is a good idea."

"Oh, you are thinking about it for the whole population," he said. "But I am thinking it is good for the individual."

"No," I said, "I'm talking about it not being good for me. I don't want the test."

We went back and forth and the volume of our comments rose. And then it dawned on me, this guy is about to cut on my crown jewels, it's probably not wise to annoy or aggravate him much more. So, I relented. Several weeks later when he called with the test results, I said, "You got that test for yourself, I don't want to know the result." And I hung up immediately.

Two other times I got the test as part of the medical screening to get life insurance policies. And the last time I did not know I was getting the test until the results came back. The health system where I get my routine care was conducting one-time "routine screening" that included hepatitis C and the human immunodeficiency virus (HIV). All three tests were done without patient consent. Each time I was mad that I got a test that I believe men without symptoms should not get. Other people and, more importantly, official guideline bodies disagree with me. That means this is not open and shut the same way colon or cervical cancer screening is. So it is important to understand the situation in order to make an informed choice.

Let's begin with basic data. The average age of diagnosis of prostate cancer is 67. At that age, an average US male will have 16.5 more years of life. Prostate cancer is almost unheard of in men under 40. About 1 in 8 men will be diagnosed with prostate cancer over their lifetime, but much fewer (just 1 in 44 men) will die from it. Importantly, 5 years after diagnosis of prostate cancer, over 97% of men are still alive. That means that the vast majority of men with prostate cancer will die *with* prostate cancer, not *of* prostate cancer.

Most importantly, in studies that have used PSA testing to screen men, after 15 years only a very small number are spared a prostate cancer death that would have happened. PSA screening reduced prostate cancer deaths from 8 in 1,000 in the unscreened group to 7 in 1,000 men in the screened group—just 1 in 1,000 men was saved. As a recent paper that enrolled over 400,000 men put it: "the absolute mortality benefit was small." However, the real finding is that PSA testing did *not* reduce overall mortality—men just die at the same time from something else. Being older, men with prostate cancer tend to have other diseases—heart disease, other cancers, diabetes, emphysema. Or as one expert on this paradox of cancer screening put it: "[I]ndividuals at high risk for cancer death are also at high risk for death from other causes. While screening might be expected to lower the former [cancer risk], it would not be expected to lower the latter [risk of death from other diseases]." So, overall, PSA screening gets more prostate cancer diagnosed and treated, reduces the deaths from prostate cancer a tiny amount, but does not ultimately save lives. I really don't care what is written on my death certificate. If I die at the same time from prostate cancer or, say, a stroke, what difference does it make?

How can that be? Before around 2010, men were commonly pushed—like my urologist pushed me—to do routine PSA screening beginning at age 50. The PSA test was seen as something of a man's version of the mammogram. PSA testing reached a peak in 2008. Since then, the US Preventive Services Task Force (USPSTF) recommendations on PSA testing have changed significantly. In 2012, USPSTF flipped entirely and recommended against PSA screening for adult men. Then in 2018, USPSTF changed its recommendation once again to advise case-by-case, physician-patient decision-making for PSA testing. Now the USPSTF is revising its recommendations once again and will probably recommend testing for any man over 55 with a 10-year life expectancy, which is what many other professional societies and organizations recommend.

Why all this flip-flopping? One of the main reasons is because PSA is not a very good test. A normal PSA is below 4.0 nanograms per milliliter. Men who have a value between 4 and 10 typically go through an MRI and then likely a biopsy procedure. But it turns out that only about 1 in 4 men with a PSA between 4 and 10 actually have prostate cancer. That means that 70–75% of men who get a PSA bewteen 4 and 10 have follow-up procedures and don't have prostate cancer. You might think this is a good ratio until you consider that no medical procedure, such as a prostate biopsy, is risk free. Indeed, there can be pain, infections, and hospitalizations after biopsies.

But the low rate of undergoing a biopsy when you don't have cancer is not the reason to be skeptical of PSA. The much bigger problem is a great deal of overdiagnosis of prostate cancer. Fully 20–50% of the men who are diagnosed with prostate cancer based on PSA testing would have lived perfectly normal lives without a diagnosis of prostate cancer much less one that caused a health problem or death. This causes two problems. The first is that treatment for any cancer is not benign; it is going to cause problems. If a man undergoes surgery—radical prostatectomy—or radiation to treat the prostate cancer, he faces a small risk of death just from the procedure itself, and a real risk of living the rest of his life with impotence or incontinence. It is hard to get the precise numbers of the risk of these side effects. The surgeons and radiation oncologists always say something like: "Things are improving with modern treatments. Compared to the studies conducted years ago, the risks are going down, so you cannot rely on the published data." But even the prostate patient advocacy groups are a bit hesitant. As the Prostate Cancer UK group says: "It [is] impossible to ignore the fact that PSA testing does save lives but also—in both of these trials—leads to a lot of extra biopsies and a lot of extra diagnoses of harmless cancers."

A prostate cancer diagnosis that won't cause death and doesn't have any complications from treatment still has serious side effects. Just having the diagnosis of prostate cancer creates a lifetime of uncertainty, worry, and the hassles of periodic additional medical appointments and tests. And if there is one thing I have learned as an oncologist, there is nothing

worse for people than uncertainty and worry about whether a
cancer will recur or metastasize. It is stressful and always present even if unconscious. We tend to downplay and not "count"
the burden of uncertainty and worry, but they are very real.
And this overdiagnosis means that millions of men—and their
wives, partners, and families—worry for years, unnecessarily.

My feeling is that I don't want a high chance of overdiagnosis of harmless prostate cancer and the real risk of lifetime impotence or incontinence and worry for no lowering of
my overall chance of dying. I really don't care that my chance
of dying from prostate cancer goes down if it just means that I
will die of something else at the same time. For the real question of living longer I get no gain and only increased risk of
very unpleasant side effects now. What is the exact benefit?

But I know that many people—and professional organizations—disagree with me. And when you read this and consider the data, you might too. Therefore, if you opt to get PSA
screening, you should start at age 55 and, more importantly,
stop getting tested at age 70 or when you have less then a 10-
year life expectancy—which is certainly by 80. Then the benefits of detecting this slow-growing cancer are definitely not
worth the side effects.

There are other screening tests worth getting at least once,
depending on individual risk factors, including screening for
hepatitis C and HIV. Ask your primary care doctor which
you need, get them, then smile when you realize you aren't
a schmuck.

Pursuing personal safety is a primal instinct and of course
a central part of staying healthy and living long. When people hear about crime going up or a murder in their neighbor-
hood, they legitimately want to protect themselves and their
families. Buying a weapon to shoot the bad guys might seem

like a reasonable choice, but the data are clear: **owning a gun**—unless you are a hunter—is a schmuck move because it *increases* your risk of injury and death.

A study of over 18 million adults in California showed that having a gun in your house makes you twice as likely to die by homicide, relative to a neighbor without a gun. Paradoxically, lethal shootings were most often by a relative or friend—not a gun-toting stranger. Indeed, having a gun makes you no safer from invaders or criminals than someone down the block without a gun.

The data on gun deaths are heartbreaking. Guns account for 55% of all suicides and nearly 80% of all homicides in the United States. What's more, there are more gun deaths in the United States every year than deaths from motor vehicle accidents. Even more depressing, about 43% of firearms are stored loaded, and about half of those are unlocked. Children find them in nightstands or dressers. Tragedy follows. Irresponsibly stored and poorly maintained guns are part of the reason that in 2019, firearm deaths surpassed motor vehicle crashes to become the number one cause of death among children and adolescents.

There are plenty of other self-destructive things to avoid, especially if you care about wellness. Think opioids, cocaine, and methamphetamines—together they caused over 107,000 deaths in 2021, more than car accidents, diabetes, or liver disease.

I would be remiss to leave out the schmuckery of getting a colonic cleanse or detoxing. Cleanses have gained increasing popularity to clean out toxins and chemicals that are supposed to cause conditions such as arthritis, asthma, fatigue, and headaches, and to boost the immune system. Colonic detoxing is bunk. There is no scientific evidence that it has any medical benefits. Moreover, cleansing has real risks. Some cleansing solutions contain potentially harmful ingredients. On the less serious side, cleansing can cause cramping, bloating, and diarrhea as well as dehydration. It can also change your microbiome by removing bacteria necessary for health. Ultimately, it can cause bleeding and colon perforation, and there are reports of deaths from coffee enemas. Don't be a detox schmuck.

You might also rethink your plans to climb Mt. Everest. Ironically, the Everest death rate has improved, but it is still 1% of all climbers. (And most bodies remain on the mountain.) The older you are, the higher the death rate. The inflection point is about age 40, such that among climbers over 59 years of age, 4%—1 in 25 climbers—die. As one guide company put it: "While summit success rates have improved, with more climbers reaching the peak than ever before, the death rate remains high, particularly for older climbers and those attempting the north route." These risks are way higher than the risk of dying in BASE jumping—1 death in 2,731 jumps—or skydiving—1 death in about 100,000 skydives. (The injury rate in BASE jumping is higher—about 1 in 250 jumps.)

While there is a lot to be said for not living an anxious, fearful life and instead challenging yourself with new activities to suck the marrow out of life, there is also a lot to be said for being prudent and reasonable. I don't know about you, but a 1 in 100 chance of dying for a young person and a 1 in 25 chance of dying for a senior, only to get some fleeting bragging rights for having gone up Everest, seems like a schmuck move. While we are at it, even the lower risks of BASE jumping seem schmucky. But skydiving might be all right—that risk is reasonable and on par with intense running, like for marathons.

Whatever your commitment to wellness, start by avoiding the excessive risks of serious injury, brain damage, or death associated with these unnecessary activities. This first step is the low-hanging fruit. Though these tips may lack the flashy appeal of the latest longevity diet fad or digital device, following these simple don'ts offers the best foundation for a healthy, long life.

2

Talk to People

Cultivating Family, Friends, and Other Social Relations

My father was the least spiritual or philosophical person I have ever known. I doubt he spent 5 minutes in his whole life wondering about the existence of God. And he certainly was not preoccupied by what existed before the Big Bang or questions about whether life is actually a dream.

Conversely, Dad was incorrigibly social—the quintessential "people person." He was endlessly intrigued by and insatiably curious about people, their lives, and the experiences that shaped them. He wanted to know what motivated them, what they loved and hated, what fulfilled and frustrated them, and how they spent their time.

In any restaurant, within 5 minutes of sitting down, Dad would be deep in conversation with the people at the next table. He would ask about their occupations, their hobbies, where their family was from, and how they came to the town where we happened to be. The subjects of my Dad's sociability did not react as if it was an FBI interrogation but rather were pleased to talk with someone who took a genuine interest in them. If there weren't other people sitting near us, Dad would strike up an extended conversation with the waitress. (When I was a child, it was always a waitress. Waiters were only in highfalutin' restaurants we couldn't afford.) And if he sensed some reticence to talk about themselves, my father would switch to more neutral topics, such as what was good on the menu and what to do in the area. His social nature was always well received. One time, our casual chat with strangers at a park even culminated in an invitation to join them for a home-cooked meal that evening.

My father was always willing to help people—friends, patients, or people he just happened to encounter. He was not shy about making medical diagnoses on a bus or in a park, giving strangers some friendly advice. He would suggest that a person with a goiter talk to their physician or remark to a parent of a child with an irregular gait that a brace might be needed to straighten it out.

I feel certain that my dad's sociability was a major contributor to his long and happy life. At 92, he died peacefully, at home, in his own bed, of a brain tumor that he did not treat, having seen all of his children and many grandchildren over the previous week. And his memorial service was overflowing with former colleagues, friends, former patients and their parents, and other members of the many communities to which he belonged.

My mom is also a very social person. As a child and adolescent, I remember her as an indefatigable organizer—gathering people to attend civil rights and anti-war demonstrations or inviting them to our house to learn nonviolent protest techniques. She was also a superb listener, adviser, and helper. She was particularly good with adolescents, making them feel understood in that most dynamic and strange period of life.

Many stray friends and relatives took refuge at our home for prolonged periods of time. And I mean prolonged. One cousin stayed two years.

And my high school friends loved to come to a house where there was no judgment. Mom was constantly helping people in trouble, taking in a child from a couple who had long-term mental health issues or hosting a cousin recovering from hepatitis. Despite her current limitations with walking and hearing, she still retains her wry sense of humor and at 91 declares: "I have no diseases that will kill me." Her generous and social spirit is a key to her longevity and well-being.

My parents were the paradigmatic embodiment of Aristotle's famous idea that "man is by nature a social animal." Nearly 2,500 years ago, Aristotle acknowledged the importance of having friends and social relationships by devoting two chapters of the *Nicomachean Ethics,* his book on ethics, to elucidating the nature of friendship. Aristotle believed that embodying the virtue of being a good friend, and practicing friendship often, was one of the central pillars of being a good and virtuous person.

Many wellness and longevity enthusiasts are obsessed by exercise, diet, and sleep—the *physical wellness behaviors.* These are vital, of course. But too often they ignore the importance of family, friends, and social relations—the *emotional wellness behaviors*—which have a remarkable impact on the quality and length of one's life. And it is a dangerous fallacy that a deficit of emotional wellness behaviors can be remedied with a surplus of physical wellness behaviors. No amount of kale or number of steps or hours of sleep can replace the importance of building and maintaining good relationships for wellness and longevity. Indeed, it seems that an obsession with exercise is often pursued as a coping mechanism for loneliness. Think of the chronically friendless and lonely Travis Bickle in the 1976 classic movie *Taxi Driver*:

June 29th. I gotta get in shape. Too much sitting has ruined my body. Too much abuse has gone on for too long. From now on there will be 50 pushups each morning, 50 pullups. There will be no more pills, no more bad food, no more destroyers of my body. From now on will be total organization. Every muscle must be tight.

Or remember Alan Sillitoe's classic short story *The Loneliness of the Long Distance Runner*, published in 1959 and later made into a movie. Smith is a socially alienated, despondent, and underprivileged adolescent. After being arrested for robbery, he is sent to juvenile prison. In one of those classic battles of the haves versus have-nots, the prisoners compete against an elite private school in a cross-country race. Smith has the speed and endurance to win, but in an act of rebellion against the prison authorities, his fellow prisoners, and society more generally, Smith deliberately loses the race.

Often, among young adults, gym culture is centered around solitude. It's a mechanism to get over an ex or survive an intense boss or defy social norms. The superiority of solitude has persisted into the 21st century and undergone a rebranding in the social media landscape. The "sigma grindset" is a social media school of thought that encourages young men to equate "grinding alone" with productivity. Sigma males are "self-sufficient loners" who prioritize meditation and solitary 5 a.m. gym sessions over socializing.

This socially isolated grinding mindset is a mistake. When it comes to wellness, family, friends, and social interactions are not superfluous or "nice to haves" *but probably the most essential elements of wellness, longevity, and happiness.* The best and most interesting data come from a report with the bland, eye-glazing title The Harvard Study of Adult Development. The study began at Harvard Medical School in 1938 and was initially called the Grant Study, named for its benefactor, the Grant Foundation. The study enrolled 268 white male Harvard undergraduates, including future president John F. Kennedy and famed *Washington Post* editor Ben Bradlee. The cohort comprised sophomore men from the Harvard College classes of 1939 to 1942; about half were socially upper class and the other half were on scholarship—but all were high achieving. Ahead of its time, the Grant Study's object was to figure out what led to healthy young adult development.

Simultaneously, a Harvard criminology professor named Sheldon Glueck, who also happened to be a leading advocate for establishing the International Criminal Court after World War II, and his wife Eleanor Glueck, a social worker, initiated a parallel study of 456 12- to 14- year-old boys from poorer Boston neighborhoods. These boys were mostly from troubled, low-income immigrant families, but had avoided what was then called juvenile delinquency or engagement with the criminal justice system.

While the two studies began separately, they were combined to create the Harvard Study of Adult Development with a total of 724 white males. Subsequently, the spouses of each group were enrolled, and later their children in what is known as the Second Generation Study. Today, these data from over 2,000 individuals elucidate how childhood experiences influence wellness, aging, and happiness.

Participants have been surveyed every few years about their lives, physical and mental health, marriage, career, retirement, and wellness. Every 5 years, the participants' physicians were contacted for specific health information.

Every 5 to 10 years, the men were interviewed for more qualitative data "about their relationships, their careers, and their adjustment to aging." With about 85 years of follow-up, it is widely regarded as the longest-running study of wellness and longevity.

The conclusion: Good relationships are the single strongest predictor of both a *happy* life and a *long* life. Robert J. Waldinger, a professor of psychiatry at Harvard and the current head of the study, summarized the findings this way: "The people who were happiest, stayed healthiest as they grew old, and who lived the longest were the people who had the warmest connections with other people. In fact, good relationships were *the strongest predictor* of who was going to be happy and healthy as they grew old" (emphasis added).

Or as Dr. Waldinger puts it in his recent book *The Good Life* (2023):

> One crucial factor stands out for the consistency and power of its ties to physical health, mental health, and longevity. Contrary to what many people might think, it's not career achievement, or exercise, or healthy diet. Don't get us wrong: these things matter (a lot). But one thing continuously demonstrates its broad and enduring importance.... *Good relationships keep us healthier and happier. Period.*

The Harvard Study of Adult Development is not the only study to demonstrate that family, friends, and social interactions are the most important determinant of wellness, longevity, and happiness. There are many other long-term studies in the United States and elsewhere that cumulatively have followed hundreds of thousands of people from diverse backgrounds to identify what contributes to a long, vigorous, and fulfilling life. One of the biggest studies is the Chinese equivalent of the Harvard Study: the Chinese Longitudinal Healthy Longevity Study, overseen by a professor at Duke and Peking Universities. Like the Harvard study, the goal is "to investigate the social, behavioral, environmental, and biomedical factors and their interactions that may influence healthy longevity." Between 1998 and 2018, the researchers conducted over 110,000 face-to-face home interviews with people from middle age and up, particularly focusing on people who lived to be over 80. Nearly 20,000 participants were over 100 years old. Researchers in this study found a similarly strong association between social activities and longevity. For instance, playing cards—like mahjong rummy—with other people and participating in organized social activities were associated with a longer lifespan. Interestingly, they also found a strong association between increased social activities and diminished risk of developing functional impairments, such as needing help with dressing, walking indoors, and bathing. Most importantly, while socializing monthly or weekly helped, the study showed that participating in some kind of social activity almost every day had the most significant association with prolonged lifespan.

Another piece of evidence for the importance of family, friends, and social relations comes from the Health and Retirement Study. It involved more than 20,000 nationally representative Americans older than 50. For each participant, the researchers looked at their number of friends, the frequency of contact with them, and the quality of the contacts. With repeated interviews over 8 years, these researchers also found that friendships are strongly associated with wellness and longevity, specifically a 24% reduced risk of dying during the study period, a 17% lower risk of depression, and a

9% increase in physical activity. And don't forget, socializing improves cognitive functioning.

Nearly 40 years ago, a study interviewed and followed a random sample of more than 17,000 Swedish adults for 6 years to assess how their social interactions correlated with longevity. Even after controlling for known risk factors that shorten life—age, smoking, lack of exercise, chronic illnesses, and the like—having fewer social interactions increased the chances of dying in just 6 years by about 30%. Similarly, a more recent Australian study of people over 70 found that a greater network of friends was associated with a 22% decrease in mortality over the next 10 years.

Studies that followed large groups of people for years have shown the importance of social relationships for wellness and longevity. These findings are bolstered by the growing consensus that loneliness is deadly. Much of the data substantiating this bold claim are summarized in the surgeon general's superb 2023 report, *Our Epidemic of Loneliness and Isolation.* This report will soon be recognized as a landmark in the history of public health, as significant as the 1964 surgeon general's report on the risks of smoking. Among the highlights is a meta-analysis led by Julianne Holt-Lunstad, of Brigham Young University. The BYU researcher aggregated data from 148 studies that followed more than 3 million healthy people over time. It found that "among initially healthy people followed over time, loneliness was associated with a 26% increase in the risk of premature death, social isolation with a 29% increased risk, and living alone with a staggering 32% escalation in mortality risk." In fact, loneliness and social isolation can be as bad for your health as smoking 15 cigarettes a day. Even more worrisome is that loneliness and social isolation are greater risk factors for dying among people under 65.

Social connection has a profound impact on long-term physical wellness, even for physically healthy young people.

You might be asking yourself: What about introverts? Surely, their wellness is not going to be improved by engaging in even more social interaction. Wrong. Many studies have shown that if you are among the 25–30% of the population that is introverted, acting more extroverted—being more gregarious and engaging with other people—will make you happier without depleting your willpower or energy. As some researchers argue: "Even highly introverted individuals experience an increase in positive affect after socializing." Paradoxically, introverts "misjudge how they will feel after acting extroverted. . . . They kind of underestimate how much fun it will be to act extroverted" and socially engage. Researchers in Canada studied nearly 1,000 people during the isolation of COVID-19. They showed that even among introverts, individuals who were less lonely and got more support from family and friends were much happier. Indeed, introverts might even gain more from social engagement than extroverts. When it comes to the importance of social relations, introverts are fundamentally human, and these relations are just as important to their health.

As Aristotle understood, the social nature of human beings means that these findings are universally true; they hold regardless of sex, gender, previous health behaviors, current health status, country of residence, and even personality type.

These long-term population studies have produced overwhelming and incontrovertible evidence: Loneliness kills, while strong social relationships promote up to a 50% increase in survival. But how does loneliness kill? What is the biological mechanism by which social relationships extend health and longevity?

Several plausible biological mechanisms have been identified to explain the links between loneliness and morbidity and mortality. Social interactions change our physiology by influencing the sympathetic nervous system—the fight-or-flight response—as well as inflammation and the immune system's response to viruses.

A recent study elucidated exactly why and how loneliness can cause biological changes and poor health. Researchers looked at people experiencing social isolation and loneliness to understand how these social experiences directly influence physiology, separate from their comorbid impact on anti-wellness behaviors such as poor diet and lack of exercise. They used data from blood samples of over 42,000 people in the UK Biobank to investigate if loneliness and social isolation are associated with specific protein markers in the blood. They found that "loneliness causally contributed to the abundance of 5 proteins." And these loneliness proteins are dangerous: In the shorter term, they were linked to increased inflammation and an impaired immune response to viral infections. In the longer term, over the 14-year follow-up period, they were linked to cardiovascular disease, stroke, and mortality. This is only the beginning of research directly linking loneliness, physical health, and longevity. But the biology is already becoming clear. Feeling lonely is linked to changes in inflammation, immune system functioning, and other physiological mechanisms that in turn are associated with heart disease, stroke, and ultimately death.

This finding should be great news to everyone—it means that you can work toward improved longevity and wellness by prioritizing friendships and social relationships. Even better, it does not require short-term trade-offs for long-term benefits. Spending time with people we care about is immediately enjoyable and increases life's fulfillment. No willpower should be required: Nurturing meaningful relationships and cultivating supportive social networks make us happy right now and healthy over a lifetime. And there is an added benefit: Spending time with friends is not just good for you, but also good for your friends. You can become a lifesaver just by spending time with other people.

Unfortunately, when it comes to social connection, American society—and indeed the world—is going in the wrong direction. Despite an increasing awareness of the emotional and physical benefits of friendship and connection, Americans are becoming more isolated. We have fewer friends. In 1990, 63% of Americans had 5 or more close friends; today that figure is only 38%. In 1990, only 7% of American adults had few, meaning 0 or 1, close friends; by 2021, that number had nearly tripled to 19%. The number of people eating alone has also increased dramatically. In 2003, about a third of American meals were eaten alone. As of 2015, that number rose to over half. Sadly, breakfast, lunch, and dinner, both at home and out, have become more solitary affairs. In 1984, the movie *The Lonely Guy* portrayed dining alone as unusual and embarrassing. But responding to and encouraging the trend, more of today's commentators are romanticizing the experience of dining alone with such articles as "The Glories of Dining Out Alone" and "Why I Love Eating Alone in Restaurants." The most recent data show that 25% of Americans eat *all* their meals alone—a 50% increase in 2 decades. And it is worse among young people under 25 where dining alone numbers increased 80%. Dining alone is totally anti-wellness: "The extent to which you share meals is predictive of the social support you have, the pro-social behaviors you exhibit, and the trust you have in others."

This reduction in daily connection has been rapidly accelerated by smartphone use and was turbocharged by the isolation of the COVID-19 pandemic. But even before the smartphone and the pandemic, many opportunities to casually socialize—chats by the coffee machine at work, passing the peace at church, meeting other parents at the PTA—were fading. This is what Robert Putnam, a Harvard political scientist, famously called the "Bowling Alone" phenomenon in his landmark 1995 article and 2000 book. People were bowling more than before, but rather than doing it socially in leagues and with friends, they were doing it by themselves. Today Putnam argues that over the last 25 years, the trend toward social isolation has been "deepening and intensifying."

Nonetheless, smartphones and the pandemic made it worse—much worse. A study using data from the American Time Use Survey provides a pretty bleak summary of the situation between 2003 and 2020: "Social isolation increased, social engagement with family, friends, and 'others' (roommates, neighbors, acquaintances, coworkers, clients, etc.) decreased, and companionship (shared leisure and recreation) decreased.... The pandemic exacerbated upward trends in social isolation and downward trends in non-household family, friends, and 'others' social engagement."

For us, here and now, there is no mystery. Want to live a happy, healthy, longer life? Make and keep close friends. Unfortunately, ever since the pandemic, Americans are out of practice talking with people, making them anxious about socializing. This anxiety creates a negative self-reinforcing cycle: If anxious about socializing, people withdraw from social interactions, become less capable of meaningful engagement with others, become even more anxious about socializing, and ultimately engage with people less. The Pew Research Center found that over a third of Americans said that socializing had become less important to them after the pandemic, which in turn will make them feel more isolated and more scared of socializing. And younger Americans are almost twice as likely to report feeling lonely than those over 65.

So how can we escape this cycle? Thankfully, making friends doesn't require years of focus or practice. We are naturally social. And while this fact alone may not assuage all of our initial fears, once we get over our apprehension about rejection or disinterest, interacting with other people is psychologically fulfilling.

One of the things I learned about social relations from my father is the importance of boldness. As a kid, I was (and, to a smaller degree, still am) a bit hesitant to initiate conversations or just go up and introduce myself to new people. Many of us feel this way, sometimes without realizing it. What drives this hesitation? There seem to be two factors. One is the misperception about the costs and benefits of casual conversations with strangers, and the other is fear related to our sense of being interpersonally incompetent. Is a conversation with a stranger going to be boring and a waste of time? How should I initiate a conversation without appearing to be intrusive or a schmuck, or worse, a socially inept schmendrick? What should I say? What if the other person ignores or rebuffs me with a snide comment?

My father would answer these questions with one of his four adages about casual conversations, which he always repeated when he noticed that we were embarrassed by his social engagement.

First, "Conversations are good, be an initiator." He would observe that most people *want* to connect and will enjoy talking with you, but they are shy or, like you, worry that the other person won't reciprocate. But if you boldly assume the burden of beginning a conversation, he would argue, most people are happy to engage. As proof, he would note how willing the vast majority of people were to talk to him, and how much they enjoyed the conversation. When my father gave this advice, the data on the myriad benefits of casual conversations was nonexistent, but he intuitively knew what the research now shows: conversations, even brief ones with strangers, are fun and rewarding.

Second, "Let curiosity drive the conversation." What made it possible for my father to be a social initiator was his genuine interest in other people. I think he often tried to imagine what was going on in their heads. Doing so made it easy for him to start a conversation because he wanted to discover the secret of their lives. He frequently reminded us that he always learned something from his conversations with strangers.

This relates to his third bit of advice: "Ask questions and follow-up questions, and affirm the value of the conversation." People love talking about themselves, their family, their city, things they like. Asking questions makes the other participants like the conversation too. By asking follow-up questions, you communicate your continued interest and that you are paying attention to what the other person is saying.

My father's last adage was: "You're not so fragile. Being slighted or snubbed by someone doesn't actually hurt. And it probably has nothing to do with you but rather means the other person is having a hard time." We are all afraid of being hurt. Initiating a conversation with a total stranger invites the risk of rejection. But what is the real harm? We feel embarrassed or less worthy? My father could never understand these emotional reactions. Occasionally, his efforts to talk to someone at the next table fell flat. But he would just shrug it off, thinking something along the lines of "their loss" or "I hope whatever is worrying them isn't too serious." And when we asked him about it, he would just point out that there was no need for embarrassment. Instead of worrying about a bruised ego, he would suggest having charity. The other person was probably dealing with something serious—an urgent deadline, a distressing argument with their spouse or kid, or maybe a medical issue. After all, you will likely never see these people again, and if you did, they will simply know that you are open to conversation. While he never put it this way, my father truly believed in the motto "Nothing ventured, nothing gained."

In following these adages, he never came across as intrusive, manipulative, or calculating. Just a nice person who was interested in what other people were thinking.

My dad's adages are embodied in Katie Hafner's novel *The Boys* (2022). One of her characters is socially inept with a phobia about starting conversations. He is going to meet his girlfriend Barb's parents for the first time and is nervous. To calm him, Barb gives him advice:

> "All you have to remember is that people love to be asked questions."
> "I don't."
> She ignored that. "And people love to talk about themselves. Asking one good question is like pushing the play button."
> That second observation applied even to me, since meeting Barb. She would ask me the simplest question—"How was your day?"—and I was off and running. I delivered entire soliloquies.

Gillian Sandstrom, a researcher at the University of Sussex in the United Kingdom, writes about her experiences talking to strangers, which basically affirms my father's views:

> One of the first times I remember deliberately starting a chat with a stranger was on the subway in Toronto. It was at a time when there was a wave of amazing cupcake

shops, and this lady on the subway was carrying a beautiful cupcake. I started asking her about the cupcake, but ended up learning from her that people can ride ostriches! I was hooked. Since then I've had many adventures talking to strangers.

Enthralled by the transformative act of talking to strangers, Sandstrom shifted her entire research focus to uncovering the connection between weak social ties and wellness.

Inspired by my dad and emboldened by the emerging research, I talk to the person sitting next to me on an airplane or train to find out where they are going and why. If they act reserved—or are boring—I just go back to reading my book or working on my computer. If they engage, all the better. Similarly, at a party where I don't know anyone, I don't worry about introducing myself to strangers. I just use the tried and true method I learned from my dad: asking them questions about themselves. If it doesn't work, I just move on, likely never to see them again.

I also respond when someone engages me. I was riding an Amtrak train, and the conductor came by to scan my ticket and noticed the book on my little table, *King*, by Jonathan Eig. He asked me if I liked the book; he had not read it but was wondering if it was worthwhile. I told him a few of the things I learned about Martin Luther King's formative years, before he led the Montgomery, Alabama, bus boycott and rose to national prominence. He said he would have to read the book. A few weeks later, I knew I would be taking his 7 a.m. train up to New York, and I brought him a copy of the King book. Since his initial question, I see that conductor about once a month, and we have become good acquaintances. He told me about one of his uncles who was a civil rights activist in North Carolina in the early 1960s and how he was run out of town for his protests.

He asks me about my teaching and writing. We frequently discuss current events. I get a little burst of joy from the human connection and interesting conversation whenever I see him.

So, forget the embarrassment and don't be shy . . . be a social initiator and talk to people, from the barista to the grocery store clerk to the Amtrak conductor taking your ticket. It will make you feel better, giving you the skills to make initiating conversations rewarding and even pleasurable. Who knows, it might just lead to a few serious friendships. And all of this social connection, even with the strangers you encounter, will enrich and lengthen your life.

Loneliness is not just an American phenomenon. It is worldwide. Gallup's World Poll, which tracks many physical and psychological factors from pain to anger to stress in 160 countries, reports that 23% of people surveyed said they "felt loneliness 'a lot of the day yesterday.'" Not surprisingly, feeling lonely was associated with feeling sad, angry, and stressed. Loneliness was not uniform across the globe. Some countries, such as Denmark, Taiwan, Estonia, and Poland, have lower loneliness levels—in the 10% range. But as the researchers argue, "no country was immune to this problem."

The global reach of this trend toward loneliness suggests a larger social problem that transcends borders: the impact of technology and social media. They are strong forces, seemingly beyond our control, that make friendships harder. Each of us individually can do our part to cultivate friendships and close social relations, but that is going against contemporary currents. It would be better if our society, through urban design, work schedules, phone-free zones, and other practices, helped us connect with people.

Robin Dunbar, professor emeritus of evolutionary psychology at the University of Oxford, is one of the great researchers on friendship. He has argued that the number of friends and social relationships we are able to maintain is limited by brain capacity, in addition to time and effort. By studying different primates, Dunbar showed that group size for each species was correlated with the size of the brain's neocortex—the thin layer of cells that are the new (neo-) addition to the brain— occurring only in mammals. This layer constitutes about half the human brain's total volume and is the site of the higher-order mental functions: sensory perception, motor movement, language, executive function, and cognition. According to Dunbar, the size of the human neocortex allows about 150 meaningful relationships (the range of variation is somewhere between 100 and 250). Thus, 150 has become known as the Dunbar number. This number has been subject to a lot of scholarly discussion and argument—but what bold new claim *doesn't* inspire controversy and argument? Dunbar points to the recurrence of roughly 150 people in a variety of historical data, such as the size of the typical English village in the 11th century, as reported in the great survey of England and Wales contained in the Domesday Book of 1086. It is also the number of soldiers in a typical military fighting unit. Of these 150 people, time and effort limitations mean we tend to have to about 5 or so closest, best friends and romantic partners, 15 good friends we trust, and 50 people we would typically feel comfortable inviting to dinner at our home.

Establishing and maintaining a close friendship requires both time and meaningful, personally revealing interactions. Usually, it takes about 50 hours to establish a connection with another person—to go from "acquaintances to casual friends." But to transform that into a closer friendship—"good or best friends"— requires about 200 hours over 6 weeks. It also requires that those 200 hours be spent meaningfully. That means not just working together or sitting in the same class, but actually engaging—exchanging thoughts and opinions, confiding in each other, chatting, joking.

This is why for so many people, college friends remain life-long friends. They are the people with whom you spent hours "shooting the shit" late into the night, confiding career dreams and romantic interests. By sharing yourself, revealing your inner thoughts, feelings, fears, and aspirations, you become close to another person.

Maintaining friendships also requires time. It requires checking in once every week or two. This may seem daunting or bothersome, a chore to add to an already busy life. But even my brothers and I check in with each other four, five, or more times a week, busy and impatient as we are. How? By keeping our conversations brief. Once, when my brother called in the middle of breakfast, I was not going to answer the phone, but my wife said, "Go ahead, the calls never last more than 90 seconds." So, what we lack in duration, we make up for in frequency. In fact, these interactions can be short because they are frequent—each interaction is part of the longer conversation. Furthermore, we know each other so well we can speak in short snippets and phrases, our own brotherly jargon. Our conversations may seem incoherent to other people but we can fill in the details around the phrases. It's almost like a secret code. But when I talk with a few of my closest friends every other week or so, the typical conversation might last for 15 to 30 minutes. I often do this when I am on my way to a train station or an airport, moments that otherwise might be filled with scrolling on my phone or looking out the window. And with other friends, I email them every few days, and then we talk every few weeks or so.

To form and maintain friendships, our interactions need to be free of distraction. This may be our hardest challenge in the smartphone era. Our phones are always at our fingertips—

even when they shouldn't be. A recent study showed that beginning at age 11, nearly one-third of adolescents demonstrate addictive social media and mobile phone behavior. A 2025 study found that teens averaged over 5.5 hours of smartphone use every day—with 1.5 hours per day *during school hours*. A quarter of the teens spent more than 2 hours on their phones during school. Even in school, it's becoming harder to look beyond the screens. A rich conversation requires your mental and emotional attention. You cannot be constantly monitoring your phone or having it beep while simultaneously cultivating a deep connection with someone. In this day and age, that requires turning your phone off... or at least turning off the ringer. It also requires putting the phone away—yes, out of sight. Studies show that just seeing your phone seems to create anticipation and mental distraction, even when it is not being used.

In one study, researchers divided 520 undergraduates into three groups. All participants had their phone ringers and vibration functions off, but one group put their phones face down on the desk, another group put them in a bag or in their pocket, and the third group put the phones in another room. Then students were given cognitive tests. One test evaluated their ability to solve math problems while keeping track of randomly generated letter sequences. Another test involved solving novel problems, like completing a pattern. These tests assess mental focus and attention. Students performed worst in all tests when the phone was on the desk, next worse when it was in the bag or pocket, and best when the phone was in another room. Interestingly, the impact of the phone on cognitive function was working subconsciously because the students perceived no difference in phone-related thoughts regardless of the phone's location. The authors concluded that "the mere presence of one's smartphone reduces available cognitive capacity, even when it is not in use." Paradoxically, smartphones make us stupider.

But it is not just that smartphones influence intellectual performance—they also undermine in-person social interactions. A recent study had participants go out to dinner with friends or family. Participants were divided into two groups: One group was allowed to keep their phones during the meal, the second group was not. Those who kept their phones during dinner were more distracted and less able to connect with their friends or family. Perhaps more surprisingly, though, those with their phones also reported more boredom and less enjoyment. Though phones are marketed as entertainment, it seems that their presence actually made real interactions less entertaining and enjoyable than when the phones were not visible.

If you are or plan to be a parent, remember that your smartphone use, like screen time, can also undermine your kids' growth and outcomes. A recent meta-analysis spanning nearly 15,000 people in 10 countries found that more parental use of technology like smartphones is associated with worse cognitive and psychosocial outcomes in kids younger than 5 years old. It also showed that more tech use by parents is associated with more screen time for these young kids. Though effect sizes were small, we can all feel this. Young children are sponges, and their exploration of the world around them should not be tainted by parental screen or other tech use. Adults, limit your screen time around young ones and seize opportunities like pushing that stroller to talk to your kids and discuss what is around them.

Compelled by this research, I make my classes at the University of Pennsylvania tech-free environments. Students are forbidden from taking their phones out of their backpacks and from using laptops to take notes. I've allowed tablets, laid flat on the desk for writing notes, but I'm considering trashing those too. The results, though decidedly nonscientific, have been extraordinarily positive. Not only have exam scores improved, but removing the distraction or preoccupation of phones from the classroom has encouraged real social connection. Toward the end of the semester, I noticed students lingering after class to chat with one another, going out to dinner, and exchanging contact information. Not insignificantly—at least for me as the professor—students also gave me and my teaching assistants much better teaching evaluations than we have received in previous years. When probed about it, a few students told our teaching team directly that they were surprised to come to like the phone-free policy. Banning phones cultivated focused attention on class and higher student satisfaction—just what the dinner study suggested would happen.

I would love it if my classroom were more like the White House Situation Room, where everyone has to put their phone into a locked cubby before entering the room. Although optimal for mental focus, this would be difficult to enact. But even small environmental changes can make a meaningful impact encouraging focus and social connection.

Of course, there are instances in which social media helps people connect. It certainly helps maintain established relationships over long distances, and social media proponents claim that support found on social media can be enriching, and even lifesaving, for some LGBTQ+ youths and other marginalized individuals. Given the increasing societal and political pressures on such kids, support and social connection is valuable wherever it can be found. But these claims may be a bit misleading, since some of these youths may be using social media as a substitute for isolation rather than for friendship. Chatting about their lives and the issues they face

with friends online is likely better than chatting with no one
at all. Such "remote connections" may be good for 5–10% of
the population who are isolated and seeking connection with
sympathetic people who share certain experiences or characteristics. But even for them, it is *not* the healthiest alternative.
And it is definitely not healthy for the other 90%.

Perhaps the biggest problem with smartphones and social
connections is what economists call opportunity costs. That
phone consumes a lot of time. The hours spent mindlessly
scrolling are hours not spent forming and maintaining social
relationships. This, in turn, increases loneliness. According to
a US study cited in the surgeon general's report on loneliness
and isolation, "participants who reported using social media
for more than 2 hours per day had about double the odds of
reporting increased perceptions of social isolation compared
to those who used social media for less than 30 minutes per
day." This is scary considering that on average American adolescents spend nearly 5 hours per day on social media, and
nearly half are online "almost constantly." It is hard to argue
that if you are spending nearly 5 hours a day on social media,
you are simultaneously able to spend quality, face-to-face
time with the people you care about.

It is not just the amount of time spent, but also the quality of social interactions that has declined. One Italian study
involving nearly 150,000 people between 16 and 75 years of
age found that smartphone use reduces both the amount of
time spent with friends and "the quality of face-to-face interactions with friends." More smartphone use means fewer
meaningful friendships. A major reason is probably that social
and other digital media have caused our attention span to
plummet. Over the last 2 decades, the average attention span
has dropped from about 150 seconds to under 50 seconds. We
are less attentive and more distractable. No wonder Ameri-

cans today report less enjoyment from the time spent being with and talking with other people—we are not paying attention to each other or the conversation.

Despite its misleading name, social media is anti-social and thus anti-wellness. As some researchers summarized it, "The use of social media may detract from face-to-face relationships, reduce investment in meaningful activities, increase sedentary behavior by encouraging more screen time, lead to internet addiction, and erode self-esteem through unfavorable social comparison." They claimed that this is especially true for Facebook, which "was negatively associated with overall well-being. . . . Facebook use in one year predicted a decrease in mental health in a later year." While their 2017 study focused on Facebook, we can assure ourselves that Instagram, X, TikTok, and other social media platforms are no different. Sadly, it's also no surprise that social media is worse for those adolescents who are already fighting mental health struggles. A recent study out of the United Kingdom found that adolescents with mental health conditions spend more time on social media and are less happy with their experiences on social media compared with those without mental health conditions. Getting off social media improves well-being, alleviates symptoms of depression and anxiety, and strengthens real-life, meaningful relationships.

So what can you do to improve your friendships? One thing is to limit your phone rings and vibrations. I routinely have my ringer off and have no phone vibrations—except if I am expecting an important, prearranged phone call. Yes, I miss calls . . . but in 2 years I have never missed anything so important I regretted it. Another idea is to limit phone use. You can do this by creating phone-free zones. My mother made sure there was no taking phone calls during dinnertime. Today, my family has a rule of putting our phones away during meals, with an important exception that we might have to find a fact or piece of information to settle an argument or bet. Recently, I bet my wife there were no American males who were super-centenarians, living over 110 years of age. This was such a point of contention, we just had to settle that bet. She got up and grabbed her phone, and . . . she won. A third approach is to have a weekly phone break: to go electronics free for just one day each week. For the last 2 years, having an electronics Sabbath has been one of my New Year's resolutions. So far, I have failed to achieve it! But I am getting better, going without my phone most Saturdays of the year.

Another way to improve your social connection and to guarantee deep conversations is to walk or hike with a friend . . . without your phone in hand, of course. Spending time in a park or forest has multiple benefits—a nearly 20,000-person study found that spending 2 hours in a park or other natural environment is correlated with self-reported good health and myriad physical benefits, such as lower blood pressure and stress. Something about the combination of walking and nature often induces more personal sharing and vulnerability—and of course can be great exercise.

These suggestions are likely to help you establish, maintain, and strengthen strong friendships. And a mountain of research shows that this will increase the length, vitality, and quality of your life.

But these strong connections are only part of a rich and rewarding social existence. People also get a major wellness boost from brief and transient social interactions—the kind my father had with the people at the adjacent table and the kind I have with my Amtrak conductor. These are called "weak social ties": connections between people in close, but not overlapping, social groups. The most common weak ties tend to be with people in your workplace or social organizations—churches, synagogues, or mosques, PTA groups, or sports leagues. Purposely cultivating routine weak social ties into your everyday life can improve your wellness, too.

A growing body of research shows that instead of making the purchase of a morning cup of coffee an instrumental, impersonal transaction—the kind we might have with a vending machine—making it a brief intentional human-to-human interaction is more fulfilling. Researchers had people making a purchase at a coffee shop smile, make eye contact, and exchange a few words with the barista. These mini-conversations generated consistently positive emotions and more connection than the buyers who were told to avoid any unnecessary interaction. Another study of over 60,000 people in Turkey and the United Kingdom found that even more minimalist interactions, such as saying hello or thanking a cashier at a bookstore, produced greater life satisfaction. A different study showed that having more of these day-to-day interactions was linked to a greater sense of well-being. And a Japanese study found the same thing. As one group of researchers noted, "[H]aving conversations with strangers ... as well as simply greeting and thanking ... predicted greater life satisfaction."

I recently had one of these transitory interactions. On one of those polar vortex days, I was riding up the elevator in my office building with my bike. A woman got on and rather than pass the time in silence, she said, "That's daring, riding a bike in such cold weather." I responded, "It was stupid too, since I forgot my gloves and my fingers are frozen." She laughed and told me that I wouldn't do that again. And then the doors opened at her floor and our interaction ended. But those few words gave me a bit of a bounce for the rest of the day.

A study in British workplaces tested different approaches to improving employee wellness. All that stuff employers are trying, from resilience training and stress management to relaxation, coaching, and sleep apps proved worthless. They generated no improvement in employee well-being. But one intervention *did* unexpectedly improve employee wellness: "Volunteering is the only type of intervention to suggest benefits for workers' well-being." Why? It is engaging with other people, even for a short period of time, that improves wellness, not the narcissism of getting into your own head through mindfulness, relaxation, and the other individual-focused interventions. According to the researchers, volunteering gave workers a sense of belonging. That is, volunteering with other employees enhanced "social resources, rather than psychological skills," and the social connections proved "more effective for improving workers' well-being."

There are two interesting things about the link between these weak social ties and well-being. One is that they are bidirectional. Talking to a stranger is good for you *and* for the person you are talking to. Both people gain. Taking the initiative is not only beneficial to you, but an act of generosity. Aristotle would approve, arguing that you can be virtuous just by asking someone a question to spark a conversation or making an empathetic comment about bicycling in the cold. The second important point is that the benefits seem to be mediated by a sense of belonging and engagement with another person. These brief social interactions seem to reduce a sense of being ignored, overlooked, and excluded. Greeting and thanking can make both people feel connected, "seen," and appreciated.

This suggests that one way to improve your social connections and thus wellness is to engage and talk to people as you travel, shop, and go about those otherwise mundane activities of daily life. As one researcher put it: "Taking the steps to practice chatting with those you encounter as you go about your day can pay off. It can make you feel better, boost your mood, and even stave off loneliness." And it can help other people in the world. That corny bumper sticker—"PRACTICE RANDOM ACTS OF KINDNESS"—could be right, but in a surprising way. Be social. It makes everyone healthier and happier.

3

Expand Your Mind

Staying Mentally Sharp

In 1776, at the ripe age of 70, Benjamin Franklin sailed for France to be the first ambassador for the newly formed United States of America. His main objective was to persuade the French to financially, diplomatically, and militarily support the fledgling nation against the world's biggest superpower—and France's sworn enemy—Great Britain. He was largely successful. The French loaned the US government money and eventually supplied military aid. Indeed, in 1781, the French admiral de Grasse sailed his fleet with over 3,000 French soldiers to the Chesapeake Bay to assist in attacking the British. His ships then blockaded the British fleet from reinforcing Lord Cornwallis's troops. This move ultimately helped make possible George Washington's victory at Yorktown that ended the Revolutionary War.

Still in France, Franklin then negotiated the 1783 Treaty of Paris, rejecting the British offer of autonomy for the 13 colonies to remain in the British Empire. Ultimately, he secured British recognition of American independence, the evacuation of British forces, and fishing rights in Newfoundland waters.

While securing the international position of the United States, Franklin was simultaneously securing his place as one of the world's greatest inventors. Before sailing back to the United States in 1785, at the age of 79, Franklin invented bifocal glasses and devised a new sea anchor to hold ships during rough weather.

In the summer of 1785, after nearly 10 years in France, Franklin sailed back to Philadelphia, his eighth and final crossing of the Atlantic Ocean. On his voyage back, Franklin did not sun himself on the deck while sipping rum cocktails. Instead he continued to observe, theorize, and engage. He mapped the temperature, speed, and position of the Gulf Stream. His work improved the speed and efficiency of commercial shipping and mail delivery between America and Europe.

Upon his return to the United States, Franklin neither retired nor remained idle. Within months, he began a home improvement project that included two additions: a large dining room to host social functions and a library to house his vast 4,000-book collection. These rooms inspired Franklin, at the age of 80, to devise further inventions, including a chair with a hidden step ladder in the underside of the seat and a special grasping arm to take books down from the high shelves of his newly built library.

His 81st year, 1787, was one of his most productive. An inveterate builder of institutions and communities, Franklin helped found the Society for Political Enquiries and became president of the Pennsylvania Society for Promoting the Abolition of Slavery. In May, he became one of Pennsylvania's delegates to the Constitutional Convention, at which he successfully argued against having a property qualification for voting or holding office. He was also an integral part of the Great Compromise, proposing that representation in the House be proportional to each state's population and representation in the Senate be equal by state. Finally, he wrote one of America's greatest speeches. His closing remarks to the convention were just 713 words, but like other famously short speeches in American history (think Lincoln's Gettysburg Address and John F. Kennedy's inaugural address), Franklin's remarks eloquently called for respecting the opinions and judgment of others and the necessity of compromise. He also noted the importance of a unanimous endorsement by the delegates of the convention "for the Sake of our Posterity." (While Franklin wrote the speech, he did not deliver it. He was a skilled writer but not a particularly good public speaker.)

In 1789, Franklin signed the first letter to Congress calling for the end of slavery and in February 1790 sent another petition to Congress to end slavery and the slave trade. The very last article he wrote, "Sidi Mehemet Ibrahim on the Slave Trade," satirized slave owners' various justifications for slavery. It was published March 25, 1790, in the *Federal Gazette*. Less than a month later, at the age of 84, Franklin died peacefully at home. Over 20,000 people attended his funeral procession. He was honored and celebrated not just by Philadelphia's ruling elite and the Anglicans and Episcopalians, but also by those who were marginalized in 18th-century America: Catholics, Jews, African Americans, and Native Americans.

Franklin's constant intellectual engagement is the model for life—staying mentally sharp right until the end. What were the fundamental ingredients to his mental engagement? Franklin was endlessly curious—always trying to understand the secrets of social and natural phenomena. He was inventive—devising tools and processes to make human life better. He was socially engaged—maintaining correspondence with over 1,000 people and collaborating with friends and acquaintances to create institutions to improve society. He was principled—advocating for values and policies that he thought were important to human life as well as the success of the United States. Most importantly, he recognized his own fallibility. Indeed, one of his most impressive virtues was his constant openness to personal growth and improvement. He acknowledged that he had prejudices, shortcomings, and failings while also recognizing his own potential to improve and learn from others. As he said in his address to the Constitutional Convention:

> For having lived long, I have experienced many Instances of being oblig'd, by better Information or fuller Consideration, to change Opinions even on important Subjects, which I once thought right, but found to be otherwise. It is therefore that the older I grow the more apt I am to doubt my own Judgment and to pay more Respect to the Judgment of others.

Franklin is the paradigm of how to "suck out all the marrow of life."

The one thing people dread more than dying itself is the possibility of losing oneself to mental decline and dementia. For me, I know that being physically healthy but mentally impaired would be the worst of all worlds. I would rather be dead than have a healthy heart, lungs, kidney, and liver without the ability to think, read, or engage with my family.

Yet as we age, our mental capacities inevitably deteriorate. Our brains literally shrink, which in turn causes functional declines. But it is important to recognize that cognitive decline does not happen all at once—in fact, different brain functions tend to go at different ages. Fortunately, as we age there are certain mental functions that are very well preserved. The classic example is *crystallized intelligence*, which is knowledge accumulated over a lifetime and consolidated in the brain's neocortex as long-term memories. If you know words like *desuetude* or *logorrhea* or *philippic* now, they will remain as you age. Your vocabulary stays with you, so older people will still win at Scrabble. So, too, do other kinds of knowledge that we accumulate over time and repeatedly use, such as a spouse's birthday, your own phone number or home address, or the sound of a favorite piece of music. Indeed, just 5 days before my father died, I was wheeling him in a wheelchair down the block. I played Bach's Brandenburg Concertos on my cell phone, one of my father's favorite pieces of music. Within just the first few measures, he told me which concerto was playing and how much he loved it.

Similarly, as we age, we retain overlearned skills—tying our shoelaces, riding a bike, typing on a keyboard, driving to work, singing a familiar song. Over decades, such information and routines have been well imprinted on the brain's cortical circuitry and therefore fade slowly. This crystallized intelligence is essential in practicing good judgment and reducing mistakes in situations that are similar to prior experiences.

Unfortunately, the other kind of intelligence, *fluid intelligence*, declines with age. Fluid intelligence is the complex ability to think critically, reason about novel or unfamiliar problems, and develop new skills. It is critically important to learning. Fluid intelligence requires specific brain functions. The brain's processing speed—how fast the brain can perform cognitive functions and respond, often with a physical action—begins to decline in our thirties and continues to deteriorate throughout life. Working memory, which involves temporarily remembering and manipulating a limited amount of information, also declines with age. This is probably why older people have a harder time calculating a 20% tip in their heads or recalling the name of a new place. Finally, there is an age-related decline in the brain's ability to learn and form new memories. Fluid intelligence requires brain plasticity, which is the ability of brain cells to form and reinforce new connections by putting the information that was temporarily acquired during the day into longer-term memory.

The simultaneous maintenance of crystalized intelligence and loss of fluid intelligence can help us understand our experiences with aging friends and family. For example, retention of vocabulary and certain frequently reiterated competencies is a major reason many people with mild or even moderate Alzheimer's disease can go about their usual routines without family and colleagues detecting their mental decline. Indeed, it probably is also why people claim that "Aunt Sally is 93 and sharp as a tack." While it is certainly possible that Aunt Sally is like Benjamin Franklin, it's far more likely that the family's engagement with Aunt Sally is focused on familiar issues that rely heavily on her crystallized intelligence. She is able to tell well-known stories, shop at familiar stores, bake her favorite desserts, talk about old friends, and ask about her beloved grandchildren. She appears to be "sharp." But it is unlikely she is using her fluid intelligence to try, much less formulate, new recipes, visit unfamiliar locales, or discuss new books or movies.

Concept formation, cognitive processing speed, mental flexibility, and critical reasoning all decline with age. And they appear to decline early, beginning at about age 45, with the decrease accelerating with age. This inevitable decline is the bad news. But there is good news too. Like all body functions, people lose mental abilities at different rates. The decline in our mental abilities lie on a spectrum, and some of us are outliers. There are the Benjamin Franklins among us, with great brain plasticity, working memory, mental flexibility, concentration, and reasoning skills preserved well into old age. But this really is exceptional. And despite a tendency to delude ourselves into thinking we are that person, it is more than likely that we are not. Our cognitive functions are going to decline as we grow older.

But don't despair, for here is the best news: We are not helpless in the face of the dreaded mental deterioration of aging. While we cannot retain the brain power of a 30-year-old forever, we can adopt—and adopt as early as possible—the right behaviors that help forestall this mental decline. While there are factors outside of our control, like genetics (the *APOE* gene) and some parts of our environment, that can increase the risk of early-onset Alzheimer's, there are also activities and habits that we can all adopt to slow cognitive decline and postpone the development of dementia.

There is a widespread theory that brain functioning—and therefore decline of brain functioning—is affected by two key factors: how much mental function you have when the decline begins and how quickly or slowly you're losing it. That first element, how much you're starting with, is called cognitive reserve. This concept is somewhat ambiguous, but the essence is that starting with a strong foundation of robust brain connections can protect against the inevitable decline in cognitive functioning. This higher baseline of greater and more diverse brain power essentially can delay the onset of noticeable cognitive impairment.

The second element, how quickly or slowly you're losing it, is called cognitive maintenance. The idea conceptualizes brain function like muscle strength or endurance: you "use it or lose it." In practical terms, this means that you can delay the age-related onset and speed of cognitive deterioration by "exercising" your brain. You should start this neural boot camp right now—even as you read this. Avoid spending too much time on passive activities like watching TV shows, movies, and sports. Also avoid repeating the same activity over and over, like doing crossword puzzles or Wordle or doomscrolling. It is not that these activities harm your brain; it's just that they don't enhance the breadth of its function. These activities "exercise" the same specific areas of the brain over and over, like reinforcing vocabulary that is already well preserved. But they do not engage a broad variety of mental functions. Importantly, prevention is the best approach. Don't wait until the forgetfulness becomes too much to ignore. That is way too late. The earlier you establish, reinforce, and strengthen new neural connections, the better. Intentionally trying new things that use different mental functions in midlife—or before—is key.

Among other things, the notion of cognitive reserve suggests that education level is an important element of long-term cognitive health. Many Americans measure the value of education by its financial return, but there are important mental returns too. Like funds in a retirement account, accumulating a reserve of brain function can protect from the inevitable losses that occur with aging. Education allows you to invest in this reserve by building the variety and strength of brain cell connections. These days, many prominent individuals are denigrating the value of education, especially college education. Putting aside the irony of hearing highly educated people with multiple degrees from elite institutions bashing higher education, there is a danger in degrading education when it is one of the best ways to enhance cognitive function into old age. Researchers have noted that the higher a person's educational attainment, the more likely they will have well-preserved cognitive functioning as they age. As one international review article points out, "A person with more education will, on average, perform better in old age than a person with less."

It is important to note that this link between education and prolonged cognitive ability is still controversial and not definitively established. One hypothesis is that educational attainment is only a proxy measure of other factors that improve brain function, given that higher education is strongly associated with higher income, better food, and other factors that may slow mental deterioration. Yet, studies where researchers control for the effect of income still find an association between education and better mental functioning into old age.

Thus, an equally compelling hypothesis is that more educated and intellectually enriched people start aging with higher levels of cognitive functioning—higher cognitive reserve. As a student, taking that biology or coding class, reading Dickinson and Tolstoy, or learning about the Renaissance or the Revolutionary War is not only enlightening—a deep value in itself—but also forces our brains to literally make new associations and connections between the brain cells.

While these brain connections do not eliminate age-related mental deterioration—indeed, evidence suggests that, on average, educated and less educated people lose brain functioning at about the same rate—education enhances our initial cognitive reserve. A well-educated person starts at a higher level of cognitive function, allowing the impact of the decline and the onset of cognitive impairment that noticeably affects functioning to occur at a later age. That is, impairment may happen, but the timing of impairment might be pushed from the 60s or 70s into the 80s or 90s as a result of a higher starting point. And those years are worth a lot. As the researchers write, "[I]t will take the individual with more education longer to reach a lower threshold of cognitive functioning at which he or she is considered functionally impaired and receives a dementia diagnosis." Study now, and your education will help keep your mind working well later in life.

So we've established that education earlier in life is important for establishing cognitive reserve for later in life. But there is also the benefit of being curious and keeping mentally engaged throughout life. Taking continuing education classes, participating in book clubs, or learning to view and appreciate the nuances of paintings are the kinds of things that can help keep your mind nimble as you age. That is cognitive maintanence.

Another proven method to delay cognitive impairment is to take up new and challenging activities—hobbies or what the experts dub "novel information activities." For example, learning a new language or playing a musical instrument can help maintain mental acuity into old age. Learning to speak Italian and playing the piano are complex activities—they involve vision, hearing, processing of unusual words or musical notation, making appropriate muscle responses with fingers and the mouth, and more. These complex demands on the brain keep people mentally sharp. However, establishing lasting neural connections requires prolonged and consistent effort. Just dabbling in a new language or taking a one-off guitar lesson is insufficient. Like any behavior change, it takes consistent effort with these hobbies and activities to create new connections in the brain. Conversely, doing the same type of thing over and over—like crossword puzzles—helps only one kind of pathway but not a wide variety of mental functions. If you enjoy your daily crossword, feel free to keep it up! But make sure to also add diverse and challenging new activities to your routine.

One fun and approachable way to introduce a novel information activity to your life is trying new recipes and techniques in the kitchen. Cooking requires complex mental and physical engagement, especially if you try unfamiliar dishes or ingredients. Regularly cooking new recipes can keep you cognitively sharper longer, and of course you get the added wellness benefit of eating nutritious food. So fire up that stove, drizzle olive oil in a pan, and whip up a delicious new dish. Then, invite friends over to share it. A wellness trifecta.

Many of the other wellness activities also protect mental faculties and reduce the incidence of dementia. It turns out that almost everything recommended in this book is good for slowing cognitive decline. Avoiding reckless behaviors, eating well, sleeping well, exercising regularly, and engaging with friends are all associated with delayed brain deterioration.

We know that football, rugby, hockey, and boxing are bad for your brain. They can cause chronic traumatic encepha- lopathy (CTE)—aka punch-drunk syndrome—the progres- sive brain disease that interferes with mental functioning. And the more head smashing you do in sports, the worse the brain impact. A Boston University study of deceased hockey players showed that those "with longer careers not only were more likely to have CTE, but they also had more severe dis- ease." Want to keep mentally sharp into old age? *Don't smash the noggin.*

Curious about what will make your brain power decline faster? First up on the list is consumption of those sweet, nonnutritious, ultra-processed foods—sugary cereals, frozen pizza, white bread, margarine, fruit-flavored yogurts, cook- ies, and chips. Not only have ultra-processed, packaged foods been linked to depression and anxiety, but they also have been linked to faster cognitive deterioration. A recent study fol- lowed nearly 11,000 Brazilians aged 35 to 74 for 8 years. At the start, middle, and end of the study, researchers tested the participants' executive functioning, a key aspect of fluid intelligence that includes verbal fluency, visual search, and mental flexibility. Simultaneously, researchers recorded each participant's food consumption with a food frequency questionnaire. The key finding was that people who ate ultra-processed foods for 20% or more of their calories had a 25% faster rate of decline in their executive function compared with people with low consumption of ultra-processed foods. If that is not scary enough, the researchers found that people under 60 who ate a lot of ultra-processed foods showed "a faster global cognition decline." How common is ultra-processed food in your diet? It varies by country. On average, nearly 60% of all calories for American adults come from ultra-processed foods. And worst of all: Nearly 70% of the calories children consume are from ultra-processed foods. Indeed, the big food corporations have taken over the baby and toddler food industry, promoting, for example, fruity-flavored yogurts filled with added sugar. Most Americans are currently eating their way to being less mentally sharp sooner as they age.

This Brazilian study was confirmed in an analysis of all the studies of ultra-processed foods and mental functioning, which included over 850,000 people. These researchers showed that after controlling for age, socioeconomic status, and known risk factors like smoking, "High UPF [ultra-processed food] intake is associated with dementia suggesting that ultra-processed diets could contribute to cognitive impairment."

Another important factor that impacts mental sharpness and contributes to wellness more generally is sleep. We know that getting sufficient sleep is key to creating long-term memories at any age, but mounting evidence suggests that the quality and duration of sleep through middle age can influence the likelihood of developing dementia. Though this connection is yet to be definitively established, researchers have found a strong association between persistent insomnia or insufficient sleep in a person's 50s and 60s with the eventual development of Alzheimer's and other dementias. Other studies have found an association between even small reductions in deep sleep with increases in the likelihood of developing dementia.

A slightly more controversial method to forestall the decline in mental functioning is exercise. Some studies suggest that habitual exercise enhances short-term and, more importantly, working memory. In 2024, researchers at RAND released a report on predictors of dementia in the United States, using 20 years of data from the Health and Retirement Study, which followed a nationally representative sample of over 50,000 people. The study measured 181 potential predictors of dementia, from sociodemographic characteristics to physical and mental health to education, work, and retirement timing. They found that "exercising (as measured by) light and moderate physical activity) is the strongest predictor of dementia incidence in both sexes.... [There are] large differentials between those who never exercised and those who exercised at least sometimes."

Conversely, multiple studies have found no impact of exercise on mental functioning or dementia. The Whitehall II study began in 1985 with over 10,000 male and female British civil servants ages 35 to 55 with diverse social backgrounds and jobs, from clerical work to top managers, to explore how psychosocial factors contributed to heart disease and diabetes. With interviews and cognitive tests being administered to the same cohort for nearly 3 decades, the study found no association between physical activity and 15-year cognitive decline. The Whitehall II researchers hypothesized that other studies got the direction of causality wrong. It is a decline in mental functioning that triggers a decline in physical activity, not the other way around.

Despite their negative results about exercise, the Whitehall II findings about the overall connection between physical and cognitive health are compelling. The association between chronic disease, such as heart failure, diabetes, high blood pressure, or kidney disease, and dementia is robust. Interestingly, the timing of disease onset matters; earlier onset of multiple chronic conditions is associated with a greater risk of dementia. Individuals with 3 or more chronic conditions at age 55 were about 5 times more likely to develop dementia than those with 0 or 1 chronic conditions. The researchers summed up all the evidence in a memorable way when they wrote: "There is emerging consensus that 'what is good for our hearts is also good for our heads,' making aggressive control of behavioural and cardiovascular risk factors as early as possible key targets for clinical practice and public health"—a critical intervention to slowing down mental deterioration and dementia.

Finally, social relationships are also important for preventing or delaying dementia. The Whitehall II researchers also assessed the social contacts of their 10,000 participants at six different times beginning at ages 45 and 55 and then followed how their cognitive function changed over the next 14 years. The main finding was that "more frequent social contacts at age 60 was associated with lower dementia risk," independent of other factors that might influence the development of dementia, such as sex, socioeconomic status, education, marital status, and employment. They also found that the key was social contact with friends rather than family, maybe because family interactions were more routine, while engaging with friends required more cognitive effort or "novel information activities" that are important to maintaining cognitive function.

————

To stave off dementia, don't retire. That is probably my most controversial recommendation when it comes to slowing cognitive decline and staying mentally sharp.

Retirement is a major shift in a person's life—a shift that many celebrate as the beginning of a well-deserved rest. However, many of the changes that accompany retirement are counterproductive to wellness and healthy aging. For many, work is a mentally engaging and challenging environment. It requires meeting and talking to new people and collaborating with others, learning new skills, and keeping a schedule. Other people depend on us at work, which may make us try harder and perform at higher levels than we would alone. All of this requires using your brain. The hypothesis that retirement is bad for your brain function goes back to the "use it or lose it" theory. Unless the brain is processing, its functionality fades. Engaging in mentally challenging or stimulating activities at work keeps the brain active. Or as two researchers argued: The "unengaged lifestyle" of retirement dramatically reduces the need to use fluid intelligence.

Studies on retirement and cognitive deterioration present a wide range of conflicting conclusions. Experts can find a study to support pretty much whatever angle they want. One recent comprehensive review of all the studies examining the association between retirement and mental functioning concludes: "Five studies revealed mixed findings regarding the relationship between retirement timing and cognitive decline, with reported positive, negative and null associations. In contrast five studies found that later retirement age reduced the risk of dementia." There are many differences in the methodology of these studies and no consensus. My review of the data suggests that "working is beneficial for well-being and health," and thus retirement is at best neutral with regard to mental functioning, but probably accelerates memory decline, cognitive impairment, dementia, and even mortality. An important nuance is that the impact of retirement is also likely dependent on personal factors, namely, the cognitive demands of one's job and how a person spends their new postretirement time.

In my view, one of the most powerful studies comes from the RAND think tank, which used country-level data to investigate the relationship between the proportion of people who were working as they aged from their 50s into their 60s and cognitive outcomes. Those countries in which more people stopped working between their 50s and 60s had greater population declines in memory and mental acuity. Indeed, countries like Belgium and Austria, where social and tax policies encourage early retirement, saw a much greater drop in cognitive performance than countries like the United States, Denmark, and Switzerland, where the majority of workers continue to be employed into their 60s. Thus, retiring at younger ages appears to be bad for the brain. Or put a more technical way: "Retirement causes a decrease in a person's cognitive ability relative to staying in the labor force." Similarly, this RAND study of 50,000 people found that people who never worked, worked less than 10 years, or were fully retired had higher risks of developing dementia. All of these studies suggest that the "use it or lose it" idea is right and that not working (retiring) is bad for mental functioning.

The Whitehall II study had similar findings. Researchers followed nearly 3,500 civil servants for up to 28 years—14 years before and 14 years after retirement. Before and after the participants retired, researchers administered tests of memory, abstract reasoning, and verbal fluency. As expected, there were declines in all these cognitive functions related to aging—whether people were working or not. However, memory declined 38% faster after retirement. The good news is that reasoning and verbal fluency did not decline faster with retirement.

There are some studies that come to a slightly different conclusion. For instance, one study from researchers at the University of Padua, in Italy, administered the same memory test over several years, both pre- and postretirement, to participants across 11 European countries. They found that memory declines with age and that retirement at the statutory eligibility age had a "long term detrimental effect on cognition . . . [but is protective] for people who retire on an early retirement scheme." This finding is a bit counterintuitive. For those that retired at the regular statutory eligibility age, retirement accelerated mental decline. But those who retired early, and thus had longer retirements, did not see the same rate of decline—in fact, retirement proved "protective." A similar study from Norma Coe, a colleague of mine at the University of Pennsylvania and an expert on the health of older Americans, reports no impact of retirement on word recall or verbal fluency, and maybe even an improvement for blue-collar workers. Mainly, these studies note that if there is a decline in mental sharpness, it occurs in the few years immediately after retirement but then plateaus. This pattern would suggest that the duration of retirement has no impact on cognitive decline.

A possible explanation for the conflicting study results of the impact of retirement on cognitive functioning may be that it is very context dependent. The kind of job a person is retiring from seems to impact postemployment cognitive functioning. While continuing to work in a cognitively demanding white-collar job appears to slow mental impairment, leaving a physically taxing and cognitively unchallenging job may be good for a person's health, including their brain health. This may help resolve the seemingly counterintuitive conclusions from the Padua study, as the researchers note that "those with the most physically demanding jobs . . . retire earlier to relieve themselves of the daily strain." Therefore, the early retirement group may not be losing daily mental engagement and stimulation when they retire. Similarly, Norma Coe also notes that "it may be easier for some blue-collar workers to engage in intellectually stimulating activities outside of their formal work settings, whereas the change in intellectual stimulation associated with retirement may be smaller for white-collar workers."

And as Coe suggests, what a person does after retirement matters for cognitive function. Giving up a job and retiring to the couch to watch TV 40 hours a week with little social engagement is likely to accelerate cognitive decline. Conversely, retiring but having strong social interactions outside of the house, such as volunteering at a local school and meeting old buddies every week for a lunch, or taking a course with your spouse on great books, or teaching your grandchildren to ice skate, is likely to maintain cognitive functioning. It may even enhance functioning, depending on your prior work setting. Financial circumstances also matter. Having the resources to regularly see your children or visit the pyramids in Egypt or take courses at the local community college will also help keep your brain working. Your individual situation and postretirement activities make a difference to how you age and retain your mental capacities.

My bottom line: To play it safe and retain more brain power . . . don't retire, especially if your job is mentally challenging and socially engaging. And if you do retire, make sure you *continue* to do things that are mentally challenging and socially engaging.

———

But let's face facts: People cannot work forever! At some point, all of us are likely to give up our jobs. Benjamin Franklin gives us a model of how to do it well. In 1748, at the age of 42, Franklin retired from being a printer. Indeed, he invented retirement for blue-collar craftsmen. During his career, he had made a lot of money from printing *Poor Richard's Almanack,* the *Pennsylvania Gazette* newspaper, and paper currency. He also created franchise printers from New England to the Caribbean. Franklin made a deal with David Hall, one of his employees, giving him the printing business in exchange for 50% of the profits for the subsequent 18 years.

After retiring, Franklin did not go to the Delaware beach to sip Madera wine. Presciently, Franklin recognized that just spending retirement on pleasurable activities instead of being mentally engaged was anti-wellness and anti-longevity:

> When I met with a man of pleasure, sacrificing every laudable improvement of the mind, or of his fortune, to mere corporeal sensations, and ruining his health in their pursuit, Mistaken man, said I, you are providing pain for yourself, instead of pleasure; you give too much for your whistle.

Idleness was not in Franklin's nature, and while he said he wanted to become a "Man of Leisure," he had a different conception of leisure.

To him, "leisure" meant not having to worry about business concerns and instead indulging in the pursuits of an active mind. Leisure for Franklin was "time for doing something useful," something that helped his fellow human beings. He intended to spend his time "to read, study, make experiments, and converse at large with such ingenious and worthy men as are pleased to honor me with their friendship on such points as may produce something for the common benefit of mankind, uninterrupted by the little cares and fatigues of business."

Franklin's main goal was to devote his leisure time to conducting electricity experiments. In the 5 or so years after he retired, Franklin made pathbreaking discoveries about electricity, naming positive and negative charge and delineating the conservation of charge. He also invented the lightning rod. For his postretirement electricity work, Franklin won the the Royal Society's Copley Medal (the 18th century's equivalent of the Nobel Prize) as well as honorary degrees from Harvard, Yale, St. Andrews, and Oxford. Indeed, it is all the things Franklin did *after* his retirement for which he is best known. The reputation he earned in retirement ensured an enthusiastic reception in France as the ambassador of the United States.

To slow cognitive decline, continue to challenge your mind. As Franklin showed, retirement ought to be planned with specific activities that will keep your brain engaged. First, ensure that you won't be lonely. Stay in touch with friends. Form a book club with them. Make regular dates to go out to a museum or a movie or a play or take a walk in the park with a friend. To avoid loneliness and be useful, you might volunteer at a school, an animal shelter, food bank, hospital, or museum. Become a Big Brother or Big Sister. Take classes on topics that interest you that you might have missed. Write an autobiography for your grandchildren.

Whatever you do, don't be a couch potato, hermit, or merely a pleasure seeker. My suggestion is to be like Ben Franklin. Ask yourself: What can I do that would be useful and helpful to the lives of others?

Finally, your brain is not going to function forever. Even the finest machines eventually stop working well—so, too, will your brain. Plan for the inevitable mental decline. Make a will so your children don't have to spend time hassling about who gets the family's 19th-century china. Talk to your family about your wishes for medical care when you can no longer decide for yourself. Let them know what you want, and don't be vague or leave big decisions to them. It is your life. Take responsibility. This also means filling out an advance care document. The "right" choices for each individual are very personal, so make sure your wishes are clear and specific to the common conditions that arise at the end of life, like dementia or chronic diseases requiring repeated hospitalizations.

Alas, aging is a fact of life. Acknowledge it rather than fight it. Don't spend all your time trying to be immortal instead of trying to be useful to others. Take the time to do the things that truly matter to you. Be open to new experiences and live a fuller, richer, healthier life.

4

Eat Your Ice Cream

Consuming Healthy Food and Drink

I had just arrived at Penn Station in New York City and was standing on the subway platform when an old acquaintance from Washington, DC, spotted me and came over. He had moved to New York City about a decade earlier, after he cashed out of his successful Internet company. We began catching up when he suddenly asked, "Zeke, you did all that health policy stuff for Obama—what diet are *you* on?"

It is a running joke among doctors that every conversation becomes a request for free medical advice. Most of the time I don't mind, but in this case, I was totally perplexed. I hadn't lost or gained weight. I hadn't developed a medical condition that required adopting a special diet. The policies I helped launch during the Obama administration, like replacing the food pyramid with an easier-to-use food plate, were intended to clarify and democratize the most reliable nutrition research. Having some kind of secret diet that I only share with tech CEOs would be against everything I stand for.

Wondering if the subway's noise had distorted what I

heard, I asked him to repeat what he had said. When he again asked about my diet, I was taken aback and stuttered, "I just eat healthily, lots of vegetables, yogurt, nuts, and no sugary sodas—"

"No, no, I mean what diet are you on?" he asked before I could finish. "Paleo, Keto, Atkins, South Beach? Raw food? Do you do intermittent fasting or cleansing?"

I began again, "I am not on any diet. I just eat good, healthy food."

Now *he* looked at me perplexed, shaking his head in disbelief. "No diet?"

You don't need to follow some special diet, and you don't need to torture yourself or scrupulously record the content of every meal to eat well. But you may need to change some of what you eat.

We Americans are fat. Over 40% of adults are obese (with 10% of adults being severely obese) and another 30% are overweight. That means that less than a third of Americans have a healthy weight. Our future is fat, too. Over 35% of American children are overweight or obese. Projections show that by 2050, over 80% of American adults will be overweight or obese. Unfortunately, our ever-increasing weight and associated poor diet has long-term health consequences. What we eat influences our risk of type 2 diabetes, heart disease, cancer, and even arthritis. And these effects are not confined to the body but extend to brain health as well. A recent study following 512 individuals over 30 years demonstrated that "healthier diets and lower [waist-to-hip ratio] throughout midlife were associated with better brain and cognitive health in older age."

This catastrophe cannot be traced back to changes in our genetics or fundamental biology. Obesity is a social disease. It became a public health crisis over the last 6 decades because we eat too much and our food contains too much sugar, salt, carbohydrates, and bad fats. Too much of our diet consists of ultra-processed foods. We are genetically predisposed to prefer this diet.

Evolutionary biologists theorize that carbohydrate- and sugar-rich foods, which are calorie dense, are appealing to us because they helped our ancestors survive food shortages and famine. Food manufacturers leveraged this innate appeal to create ultra-processed foods composed of a combination of ingredients not normally found in nature, or even in your kitchen, that make them extraordinarily high in sugar, salt, carbohydrates, and fat. These foods have few nutrients but are "energy dense," which means they are high in calories per gram of food compared with natural or unprocessed foods.

Moreover, they are "hyperpalatable," which means they stimulate the brain's pleasure centers. They take advantage of our natural reward system, making us crave them. It is difficult to stop eating them. Remember that ad for Lay's potato chips: "Betcha can't eat just one." Right, we can't, because potato chips, like many snack foods, are formulated in industrialized laboratories and kitchens with unnaturally high combinations of salt, sugar, and fats to be maximally pleasurable and therefore maximally addictive. Indeed, applying the same criteria used for addiction to drugs and other substances, researchers estimate that the overall prevalence of food addiction is 14% among adults and 12% among children. That is, the brain circuits activated by foods with high fat and sugar content—ultra-processed foods—are similar to the circuits activated by drugs and other abused substances in the brains of addicts. Then the well-honed trifecta of advertising, product placement in supermarkets, and pricing turbocharge overconsumption, making it hard for us to resist these foods that are unhealthy when habitually consumed. Food companies are happy selling more foods and making more money. But we—and the country paying for all the related ill health—are the big losers.

By some measures, nearly 60% of calories in a typical American diet comes from junk food. Consequently, average Americans consume over 3,500 calories per day—way over the recommended 2,500 per day for men and 2,000 for women. Look at images of children and adults in high school yearbooks, magazines, or other relics of the 1950s and 1960s: The person with obesity is a true outlier, not two-thirds of the pictures. Americans consume 23% more calories per day than they did in 1970, mainly by eating more grains and oils—think muffins and bagels—but less milk, fruits, and vegetables. We ate ourselves into this mess, and we are going to have to eat ourselves out of it.

As I told my acquaintance in New York, I am not a big believer in dieting. About half of all Americans have tried some kind of diet—or multiple diets. Most have eventually failed.

Everyone starts off with great motivation, putting their all into following the myriad dietary rules. Perhaps they see results: they shed pounds, their cholesterol improves, their blood pressure drops. But keeping to all those rules is overwhelming and exhausting. The diets never seem to last. Within a few months, the numbers creep back to where they started. This is true even for people enrolled in dietary research studies. When the study ends and all the supports go away, the weight comes back. It can be frustrating, demoralizing, and even unhealthy—the roller coaster of on-and-off-and-on-again weight can increase the risk of cardiovascular disease and mortality.

Failure cycles happen even with the new crop of miracle GLP-1 drugs, including Ozempic, Wegovy, and Zepbound. It is true that these drugs lead to enormous weight loss, up to 20% of body weight in the first year (about 40 pounds for a 200-pound person). And yes, this weight loss is accompanied by significant health benefits, including about a 20% drop in heart attacks, strokes, and cardiovascular deaths, improved kidney function, and fewer food and alcohol cravings. All that is huge, and I am a big fan of them. But there are problems. One is that people on GLP-1 drugs also lose muscle mass. More importantly, after about a year, most people experience a plateau in their weight loss. And since these drugs are very costly, require weekly injections, and have side effects, staying on them can be tough. Just as with diets, the majority of people who try a GLP-1 drug quit. Most studies have found 12-month discontinuation rates higher than 50%. And once people stop the injections, they return to baseline measurements in their weight, cardiovascular function, and kidney function.

Losing weight then gaining it back because of going on and off of GLP-1s (or for any other reason) is something to worry about, given results from a recent study at Vanderbilt University Medical Center. Researchers there evaluated health records of over 80,000 people spanning over 20 years and found that the roller coaster of losing weight, gaining it back, losing it again, and so on—"weight cycling"—is itself fraught with health problems. The study found that compared with weight stability, weight cycling was associated with almost 30% increased risk for obstructive sleep apnea, metabolic dysfunction-associated steatotic liver disease (MASLD), and type 2 diabetes. Even worse, cycling was associated with more than 50% increased risk for heart failure. This increased risk was independent of baseline body mass index (BMI). As the reserachers concluded, "The present findings support promoting either weight stability at high BMI or weight loss if able to be maintained to prevent the incidence of a variety of cardiometabolic diseases."

It can feel like all this effort is futile. People who have health problems caused or exacerbated by diet or excess weight, like cardiovascular disease, diabetes, or cancer, may feel doomed to a lower quality of life. So, what's the answer? Start by accepting that willpower deteriorates over time. Exercising self-control over and over while trying to adhere to a complex and rigid diet will deplete your willpower. You become exhausted fighting against temptations and cravings, return to old established habits, and eventually regain the weight. Study after study shows that expecting willpower to fuel extreme long-term dietary changes or weight loss *is* usually doomed. That is why I am averse to diets that are extreme, like eliminating all carbohydrates or sugar. For most of us, forgoing major food groups would be a huge sacrifice and demand too much daily willpower.

The secret to long-term success—that is, to eating a diet that helps you maintain a healthy weight, reduce cardiovascular disease risk, maintain steady glucose levels, lower cholesterol, and increase the diversity of your microbiome—is being selective about how you're spending that willpower. The changes need to be simple—straightforward adjustments that you can introduce as just another aspect of your routine. They need to be things that will become habitual and ultimately a routine you can enjoy.

The biggest bang for your buck comes from changing three common dietary habits. The most important step is to stop consuming foods and drinks with empty, nonnutritious calories that imperil your health: sugary drinks, snacks, and ultra-processed foods.

The number one offender is **soda**. Those 12-ounce cans of Coke, Pepsi, Sprite, Mountain Dew, ginger ale, or root beer each pack about 140 calories and about 40 grams of sugar—the equivalent of about 10 teaspoons of sugar—and they contain zero nutritional content. Just one can of soda exceeds most recommendations for daily sugar intake. No wonder that drinking 1 to 2 sodas a day increases your risk of developing diabetes by 20%.

Drink 3 of those a day and you are consuming nearly a quarter of recommended daily calories in soda alone. These sodas and other sugary drinks really are what everyone says: "empty calories." Gatorade, Powerade, and the other sports drinks might be a tiny bit better, with half the sugar and some electrolytes, but you can easily get the minerals in healthier ways.

Opting instead for the diet version of sodas, with artificial sweeteners like aspartame or sucralose, is no healthier—and might be worse by some measures. Since they lack calories, many people think that diet sodas are healthy and can help with weight loss. But lots of research shows that this sentiment is mistaken; these artificial sweeteners don't actually help with weight loss and may even lead to weight gain and increase the risk of diabetes. Recently, WHO has come out against these sweeteners. As one commentator put it, artificial sweeteners are no "free lunch."

How can these sweeteners with no calories have a negative impact? Psychologically and biologically, they reinforce an individual's desire for sweet things, which most likely leads to eating high-sugar, high-calorie foods to satisfy that craving. More intriguingly, recent research suggests they might even change your microbiome—gut bacteria—in a way that damages the body's ability to process sugar. Researchers at Israel's Weizmann Institute of Science enrolled 120 healthy adults in a study to investigate this hypothesis. For two weeks, some of the participants were fed artificial sweeteners, such as saccharin, aspartame, and stevia. The others were fed regular glucose, as a control. After the exposure period, the health and diversity of the gut microbiome and the participant's glucose tolerance (the body's ability to process sugar and stabilize blood sugar levels) were measured. Researchers found that the gut microbiome of people who consumed the artificial sweeteners was weaker and less diverse. They also found that the participants exposed to the sweeteners saccharin and sucra-lose had an impaired ability to tolerate glucose. That is, when a person previously exposed to saccharin or sucralose drank sugar water, their blood glucose shot way up—these artificial sweeteners destroyed the ability of participants to metabolize glucose in a healthy way.

In an intriguing twist, the researchers took samples of the participants' microbiomes and transferred them to lab mice. The mice were then fed glucose and their blood glucose responses were observed. The mice became like the humans: Those mice receiving transplants from a microbiome exposed to artificial sweeteners had a similarly unhealthy response to glucose. This strongly suggests that the gut microbiome is a causal factor. The upshot is that diet sodas might change your gut microbiome for the worse, making your response to sugar more like that of a person with diabetes. This causes inflammation and places stress on vital organs like the kidneys, heart, and eyes.

Both sugar-sweetened and diet sodas are bad for your health. Don't drink them. Now, when I say "don't drink soda," it is not an absolute prohibition. I hate absolute prohibitions because you are unlikely to adhere to them. *Ideally*, you should never drink these beverages. But an occasional drink—once a week or less in moderate amounts, like 8 ounces—and espe-cially used as a reward for something well done, is not going to have a measurable impact on your health. It is the daily con-sumption of a can or two of soda or, worse, a 16- or 24-ounce big gulp that causes obesity, impairs glucose response, and gives you diabetes. An occasional mocktail with the sting of ginger ale is a good alternative.

Like any well-worn habit, it is hard to stop drinking soda—the change requires lots of willpower. After all, Coke, Pepsi, and the others spend billions on developing appealing new formulations, flooding us with advertisements, and secur-ing prime supermarket and convenience store placement to entice us into drinking more soda. The only way to develop a "no soda" habit is to minimize temptation by avoiding all the triggers that make these drinks hard to resist. To do this, you may have to avoid taking your cart down the soda and juice aisles in the supermarket and avoid walking by the vending machines in your office. Prevent the drain on your willpower by minimizing the number of times you have to say no. Say no once, at the grocery store, to avoid having to say no every time you peer into your refrigerator or pantry looking for something to drink. Without the constant temptation, it will be easier to find a substitute for sugar-sweetened beverages.

Fortunately, this is one area where Americans have made real, measurable progress. The peak year of soda consumption was 2000. Since then, there has been a 25% drop. Still, we are not there. On average, Americans are still drinking 1 can of soda a day. We have to reduce that to 1 or 2 cans a week.

Even if you wean yourself off sodas and sugar-sweetened beverages, you still need to be hydrated. Drinking about 2 quarts, or 64 ounces, of liquid a day is the recommendation. Water is the best drink—no calories or other bad stuff. If you need some taste, the ideal is flavored water with a squeeze of lemon. Be careful about those commercial flavorings sold in supermarkets, as many contain sucralose and other artificial sweeteners. Other beverages, like 2% milk, have about 120 calories per cup, but unlike sodas, they contain plenty of calcium, potassium, and vitamins and 8 grams of protein. (Truth be told, I never drink milk. When growing up, my mother was fearful of strontium-90 from nuclear tests in the western deserts. She only served us powdered milk, which was colored bluish and pretty disgusting. I see no reason to waste my limited willpower on trying to down a glass of milk when water and tea do me fine.)

Coffee and tea have no calories, and even with a splash of milk, they are only about 30 calories. Plus, they have lots of benefits. For instance, a recent report showed that drinking coffee in the morning was associated with lower all-cause mortality and maybe lower incidence of head and neck cancer. Just make sure to drink your coffee and tea fairly unadorned. I remember my father adding teaspoon after teaspoon of sugar to his coffee or tea. It was as if he was adding coffee to the sugar bowl! With this approach, coffee and tea become barely better than soda. So wean yourself off the sugar. I went down from 1 teaspoon to half a teaspoon to nothing in about 2 months as my tastebuds became used to less sweetness. Similarly, beware of those Starbucks coffee drinks. One 16-ounce latte with whole milk is 220 calories—about 10% of the recommended daily calories. And those holiday specials, the Pumpkin Spice Latte or the Peppermint Mocha, can have more than 400 calories, depending on the size and the kind of milk. They are full-on meals masquerading as drinks.

After mastering your sodas and other drinks, the best thing you can do for your long-term health is to progressively reduce or change your **snacks**. Today, snacks contribute an astounding 500 calories per day in an average adult's diet. That is nearly 20–25% of total daily calories in just snacks. Often snacks are more calorific than breakfast—or we make a snack our breakfast. A single blueberry muffin, cinnamon raisin bagel with cream cheese, or chocolate croissant comes in at over 400 calories. Not only are these basically hypodermics for sugar but they also typically lack protein, good fats, fiber, and other nutritious ingredients.

Indeed, the single largest source of calories in the American diet is flour and grains, typically breads, pastries, doughnuts, and cookies, which are rarely homemade and usually contain lots of added sugar, carbohydrates, fats, and salt with little nutritional value. Since 1970, Americans have consumed about a third more grains and other cereal products in things like bread and packaged cookies.

But there is some recent good news: Like soda consumption, snacking is dropping. The big snack companies are reporting "alarming" declines in sales. For instance, General Mills sales are down 5%. Snack executives think it is driven by inflation and the squeeze on family budgets. But it is an indication that families can cut snacks—and from both an individual and a national health perspective, that is a good thing.

Want to snack? Snack on healthy items like apples, clementines, grapes, or other fruit. Or try nuts, which are probably the most nutritious snack. Even tortilla chips and salsa can be a low-calorie snack—just watch out for the salt. Again, I am not against all snacks. After all, I do love the occasional piece of cheesecake, and I love to bake cakes and cookies and tarts and pies and . . . The problem is the daily, habitual, nonnutritious snacking. Make a high-calorie, low-nutrient snack a special treat, perhaps once every other week.

Dramatically reducing the consumption of sodas and snacks could save 500 to 600 calories and 50 grams of sugar per day. That is about 30% of the calories an average American adult consumes, though only 20% of *recommended* calories, and 100–200% of the recommended daily amount of added sugar. It is said that 1 pound of body fat contains about 3,500 calories. Cutting out 500 calories per day in snacks and sugar-sweetened sodas and other beverages means you can cut—or at least avoid gaining—1 pound per week, or 52 pounds per year. You are likely to eat some of those calories in other (hopefully more nutritious) foods—and your body will readjust your metabolism—so you won't lose 52 pounds. But this quick math shows how beneficial just cutting snacks and sodas can be.

———

Beyond these snacks and sodas, there are a range of **ultra-processed foods** that all of us ought to try to eat less of or, ideally, cut out altogether.

A few years ago, I had a colleague over for a breakfast meeting. Perhaps that's unusual, but I love to cook breakfast. For a few weekends, I even had the great honor of being the chef at my own pop-up brunch restaurant in Washington, DC. I focused my efforts on serving a healthy and delicious breakfast. I made zucchini fritters and hash browns made with malanga instead of potatoes. (Malanga is a tropical root vegetable that is increasingly easy to find.)

My colleague asked me how I came to like making breakfasts. I think it began with my fatherly concern. When raising my daughters, breakfast became an integral part of the morning routine. I would get up and make sure they had a good, well-balanced meal to start the day. I made scrambled, soft-boiled, and sunny-side up eggs and omelets with toast. I made French toast, blueberry pancakes, and warm oatmeal with raisins and nuts, which they loved. I served every breakfast with fresh fruit—berries, cantaloupe, watermelon, grapefruit halves, sliced mango, kiwi, grapes, bananas, or whatever else was in season.

My colleague was bewildered, claiming that making breakfast took too much time and would overwhelm his already rushed mornings. He told me he never cooked breakfast for his children. He just popped frozen waffles into the toaster and served them with syrup.

I cringed. How could a prominent, well-educated, health policy expert who knows the medical literature serve his children frozen waffles and syrup—the epitome of junk food? High in sugary calories, low in protein and fiber. Surprised, I wanted to ask him (sarcastically) if he allowed them to drink sodas or other sugary drinks every day. Fortunately, I used all my willpower to control myself. (How uncharacteristic of me!) But this experience reminded me of the ubiquity of inattention to nutrition in service of convenience or simplicity—with unfortunate long term consequences.

It is obvious across almost every metric that two eggs and toast is a more nutritious breakfast than packaged frozen waffles. Eggs will do a better job preparing children for school and adults for work. They have fewer calories, less sugar and salt, and more protein and fiber.

Table 2: Frozen Waffles v. Two Eggs

INGREDIENTS	2 Waffles with 2 Tablespoons Aunt Jemima Syrup	2 Eggs with 1 slice of whole grain toast
CALORIES	295	216
TOTAL FAT SATURATED FAT	7 grams 2 grams	10.9 grams 3.4 grams
SODIUM	440 milligrams	280 milligrams
PROTEIN	4.6 grams	15.3 grams
SUGAR	16.9 grams	1.8 grams
FIBER	<1 gram	1.9 grams

These waffles are a great example of the other food killer: "ultra-processed food." While less scientifically precise, I prefer the label "junk food." A recent review of 45 articles on the health impacts of these junk foods found that they are associated with higher rates of heart disease, obesity, diabetes, depression, even cancer and dementia. One study followed a representative group of nearly 12,000 American adults for a median of 19 years between 1988 and 2011. They found that people who ate the most junk food, 5 or more times per day, had a 31% increased risk of dying over that time period after adjusting for sex, age, income, education, and other health behaviors.

Part of this phenomenon may stem from the fact that junk foods are energy dense—meaning they have 2 calories for every 1 gram of food instead of the normal 1 calorie per gram. A researcher at the National Institutes of Health conducted a study that fed people either ultra-processed junk food or unprocessed whole food. People who ate the ultra-processed food for just 7 days gained 1 pound more than people who ate unprocessed food.

Other than its caloric density, we don't yet know precisely why ultra-processed foods are so unhealthy. One theory is that they contain additives that increase inflammation. Another idea is that they damage the microbiome, leading to less diversity of healthy gut bacteria, which impacts toxin creation, nutrient absorption, and glucose tolerance. Regardless of the biological mechanism, we know that the lower cost, convenience, and "better taste" of junk foods is far outweighed by the dangerous associated health outcomes, including obesity, dementia, cancer, and death.

But junk food is the dominant offering in our supermarkets. Junk food includes white breads, sugary cereals, and virtually all packaged chips, cookies, and cakes. It also includes prepared frozen tacos, pizzas, and other meals. And let's not forget processed meats and cheeses—bologna, hams, salami, and American cheese. And those sugar-loaded, fruit-flavored yogurts? Also junk. Indeed, almost 60% of the calories the average American eats comes from junk food. And it's worse among the youth, who consume nearly 70% of their calories from junk foods. All told, it is estimated that nearly half of a toddler's diet is junk food.

Packaging and advertising are misleading. Even careful consumers are duped. As a parent, I would often give my daughters Pepperidge Farm Milano cookies on the ride home from school. A measly 3 cookies contain 170 calories with 4 grams of saturated fat, 10 grams of added sugar, almost no fiber, and just 2 grams of protein. Terrible. What was I thinking? Probably that they were small, marketed as "classy" and "European," and didn't seem *that* sweet. I was fooled.

And don't be tempted by Clif Bars and most of those other "healthy" power bars for breakfast or a snack. Most are only slightly better than candy bars with a helping of protein. They have a lot of calories and sugar and not much fiber—and some add in a good helping of salt. They might be a lightweight and convenient fuel to put in your backpack or jersey when you are hiking or biking, but they should not be eaten mindlessly as a daily snack. Indeed, even the fancy foreign-sounding gourmet protein bars are not better and, in some cases, worse than candy bars.

Table 3: "Healthy" Protein Bars

INGREDIENTS	Clif Bar	LaraBar	RX Bar	Hakan's Biscoff Protein Bar	Heath Bar Candy
CALORIES	280	210	210	330	210
FAT, TOTAL	9 grams	12 grams	9 grams	17 grams	13 grams
SATURATED	6 grams	3 grams	2 grams	7 grams	7 grams
SODIUM	200 milligrams	65 milligrams	260 milligrams	110 milligrams	125 milligrams
PROTEIN	20 grams	5 grams	12 grams	16 grams	<1 gram
SUGAR	17 grams	17 grams	13 grams	8 grams	24 grams
FIBER	3 grams (11% daily value)	3 grams	5 grams	2 grams	<1 gram

As Marion Nestle, among the nation's foremost nutrition scientists, has said, the aisles in the middle of supermarkets and almost all the shelves of a convenience store are a junk yard, filled with dangerous packaged foods. If you indulge, do so sparingly.

There is some important work going on to figure out if there are some "healthy ultra-processed foods"—or at least some that are not so bad. The research is important for people who don't or can't avoid the junk aisles of supermarkets, whether from habit or cost or access or lack of knowledge. But it takes too much brain power—which we all know can easily be fatigued—to remember which junk foods are really bad and which ones are not so bad. Just try to get to a place where you are minimizing the ultra-processed foods.

Those are the three big don'ts. Forswearing sugary drinks, progressively eating fewer snacks, and limiting ultra-processed junk food are three *huge* steps toward health and wellness. These alone are major achievements and will make you healthier and help you live longer.

The next behaviors are positive steps for eating well. Each is helpful—and some very helpful—for wellness. Do what you can, remembering that your willpower is limited and that small, habitual changes, especially ones you enjoy, make the longest-lasting impacts. Some of these behaviors are easier to adopt than others. But don't obsess over each one. It is not a test of your virtue, and it won't determine whether you are among the elect that God will save.

To me, the easiest small change with big benefits is to begin eating **fermented foods**. The gut microbiome is all the rage these days. I suspect this enthusiasm is not a fad, but well justified. The average human gut has about 100 trillion bacteria. That is approximately 3 times all the cells in our bodies and 1,000 times the number of brain cells. Evolution tells us that they are there for a good reason. Gut bacteria appear to play a role in many bodily functions, and an unhealthy microbiome is associated with a wide range of conditions, from obesity to chronic inflammatory diseases and even poor mental health. Consistently consuming junk food leads to a decline in the diversity of the gut microbiome and may contribute to chronic illnesses such as diabetes. An imbalance of bacteria may even account for some of the increases in cancer among young people. I believe that the microbiome plays an important role in our health. Over the next decade, we are going to learn much more about its importance in wellness and longevity.

Enter fermented foods such as kimchi, miso, sauerkraut, fermented beets and carrots, as well as yogurt, raw milk cheeses, and kefir. Kombucha is also a fermented drink, but tends to come with about 5 grams or more of added sugars and without the protein or fiber of other fermented foods.

Fermented foods have important properties, especially providing probiotics and prebiotics—the indigestible plant fibers that promote the growth of good gut bacteria. Consequently, fermented foods have been associated with anti-inflammatory effects, lowering blood pressure and improving diabetic control. Studies also show that regularly eating fermented foods reduces obesity. A recent study by Stanford researchers showed that increased consumption of fermented foods, about 1 serving per day, "steadily increased microbiota diversity [in the gut] and decreased inflammatory markers." Since the declining diversity of the gut microbiome has been linked to obesity and diabetes and the rise of chronic inflammatory diseases, this finding is very encouraging.

With no real downside and the potential for helping enrich and diversify the gut microbiome—and a cheaper price tag than packaged probiotic supplements—eating fermented foods seems like a no-brainer. So eat your kimchi and yogurt— the plain kind without the added sugars.

The second positive change for eating well is to consume more **dairy**. This is controversial, but there are many advantages. The Dutch are the tallest people in the world. On average, Dutch men are over 6 feet tall and women 5 feet 7 inches—that's about 3 inches taller than the average American man and 2.5 inches taller than the average American woman. The data prove it, but I know it from experience too: I was once at a Bob Dylan concert in a town square and everyone had to stand for the concert. I couldn't see the stage because of all the Dutch fans singing and swaying in front of me.

Interestingly, the Dutch became the tallest people very quickly. In the mid-1800s, when American men were the tallest in the world, the Dutch were among the shortest people in Europe. A change of this magnitude over such a short time means that their height today is likely not genetic but rather stemming from an environmental change. There has been a lot of speculation about why the Dutch are so tall, but one likely factor is the "voracious Dutch appetite" for dairy— milk, yogurt, and cheese. The Netherlands is the ninth-highest milk-consuming country per capita in the world. (Denmark is number one and has an average male height of 5 feet 11 inches—also markedly taller than men in the United States.)

Yogurt—excluding the sugar-sweetened fruit kinds—is highly beneficial. With yogurt, you enjoy both the benefits of dairy and the live bacteria of fermented foods. Yogurt seems to protect against weight gain, diabetes, and heart disease. In one Harvard study, it was the single most beneficial food for weight loss.

Some nutrition experts I highly respect—such as Walter C. Willett, professor of epidemiology and nutrition at the Harvard T. H. Chan School of Public Health and a former professor of mine—are more skeptical and discount widely held beliefs about the benefits of dairy, even identifying some concerns. For example, the government encourages dairy consumption to boost calcium and reduce the risk of bone fractures. But, as Willett writes, counterintuitively "countries with the highest intakes of milk and calcium tend to have the highest rates of hip fractures," suggesting that dairy consumption does not strengthen bones. Experts like Willett also worry because dairy cows often receive antibiotics and have high levels of hormones—both naturally from pregnancy and artificially from injections of bovine somatotropin, or bovine growth hormone. While they acknowledge that dairy consumption is also associated with lower risk of diabetes and colon cancer, they point out that it is linked to increased risks of prostate and endometrial cancers. They feel that all benefits of dairy products can be found by eating other foods.

These doubts and concerns are real, but they should be understood in the context of the potential benefits. Dairy products like milk, aged cheese, kefir, and unsweetened yogurt are nutrient dense and minimally processed, rich in proteins, calcium, and vitamin B_{12}. They help us grow taller in childhood and adolescence, and they help us maintain healthy body composition as we age. Because they contain large amounts of leucine and other essential amino acids for proteins, they help support muscle growth and repair, especially for the elderly, who experience loss of muscle mass. In addition, the protein and fat in dairy slow carbohydrate and glucose absorption from the gut, lowering the risk of diabetes. And dairy protein seems to make us feel full, helping us keep the pounds off.

As I mentioned, yogurt and kefir are the best forms of dairy because of the benefits of fermentation. Furthermore, the worry that dairy products are bad for the heart and metabolism because of high saturated fats seems inaccurate. A recent meta-analysis concluded that "high-dairy intake showed no detrimental effects on ... blood lipids ... and blood pressure." Indeed, full-fat dairy improved blood pressure and may increase good cholesterol. Importantly, a lot of dairy's benefits also depend on the types of foods it replaces in your diet. If substituting for processed and unprocessed meats, dairy even reduces mortality.

The upshot is this: Eat dairy in moderation. The evidence is clear that dairy—especially yogurt—is good for you, particularly if it is replacing junk food and sugary drinks. And don't worry about full-fat products. Full-fat milk has more saturated fats, but recent data show that not all saturated fats are equal. Dairy fat is protective against diabetes and does not seem to increase cardiovascular risk. So drinking milk instead of soda or eating yogurt rather than a doughnut is unequivocally good for your wellness.

The third healthful practice is to be mindful of how much **protein** you consume. Like my New York City tech friend, Americans seem obsessed with defining the next food fad. Perhaps because low-fat diets and carbohydrates are out of fashion, in recent years protein has been increasingly promoted as the new elixir of health. Some social media influencers push people to eat 200 grams of protein a day, nearly 3 times the typical recommended daily allowance for a 200-pound adult who is not an active athlete. Even if you are exercising regularly, it is about 1.75 to 2 times too much. Food and drink companies have responded by adding protein to loads of products, including water (protein-infused Trimino and Protein2o), coffee (Premier Protein Coffee), pastas, crackers . . . even alcoholic drinks (Protochol Beverage's Spiked Protein drinks with 8% ABV in 16-ounce cans). As one commentator put it, "Protein is becoming the new 'organic.'"

What to make of all this valorizing of protein? In short, we shouldn't obsess about it. Ignore these sky-high protein recommendations, which dramatically overstate how much protein you need to consume. The good news is that the majority of Americans already meet or exceed the amount of protein needed. The recommendation from a myriad of experts and professional bodies is 0.75 to 1.0 grams per day per kilogram of weight, or about 45 to 70 grams of protein daily for adult women and 55 to 90 grams for adult men. Two exceptions: First, people over 60 should eat more protein each day—1 to 1.2 grams per kilogram of body weight, or 70 to 85 grams per day. As we age, we lose muscle mass. To maintain lean body mass we need to eat more protein. And second, if you are doing more endurance-type exercises—say, running a marathon or doing the 20 bridges swim around Manhattan—or recovering from a major health condition, you will need more protein to help your body recuperate, about 1.5 grams per kilogram.

It is easy to estimate how much protein you get. Almost all protein foods have about 6 to 8 grams per 1 ounce or 1 serving. Consequently, it is easy to consume 70 grams of protein per day. Just try 2 eggs and 1 single serving container of Greek yogurt at breakfast, and you are almost halfway there. Add in some nuts, beans, or cheese as a snack, and you are eating 70 grams a day with no effort and little thought.

Table 4: Protein in Various Foods

Food and Amount	Protein
1 ounce beef or chicken	7-8 grams
1 ounce fish, like salmon	7 grams
1 egg 1 egg white	6 grams 4 grams
1 ounce almonds (¼ cup or 30 almonds) 1 ounce peanuts	6 grams 9.5 grams
1 ounce cheese	8 grams
1 container (5.3 ounces) Greek yogurt 1 container (5.3 ounces) regular yogurt	15 grams 8 grams
½ cup kidney beans	7 grams
½ cup lentils	12 grams
½ cup quinoa	4 grams

Not all protein is created equal. There are 20 amino acids that make up the proteins in our bodies. These proteins are not only necessary to build and maintain muscle—they also support immune health and tissue repair and promote normal functioning of vital organs. Surprisingly, the human body does not make 9 of these amino acids. And the one we really need—the one that really promotes health—is leucine. Indeed, leucine is kind of a miracle molecule. It is key to building and repairing muscle, wound healing, and regulating protein synthesis throughout the body. It also induces insulin secretion to regulate blood sugar. And maybe most surprising of all, leucine also helps with appetite control and thus weight control.

For such a vital component of the body, it is surprising the human body cannot manufacture leucine. You have to eat it.

That is why it is called an *essential* amino acid—it is both necessary for the body and must be consumed, making it *essential*
in your diet. The recommendations for how much you need to
eat are all over the place. One set of recommendations calls
for about 3 grams. Others suggest 5 grams, and still others
suggest about 7.5 grams of leucine per day. About 10% of protein consumed per day should be leucine. And since the elderly
need more protein, they need more leucine too.

The best source of leucine is animal muscle. For instance,
4 ounces of beef will get you about 1.7 grams of leucine,
chicken breast about 2 grams, and salmon about 1.5 grams.
But there is plenty of leucine in eggs as well as dairy products
such as milk, yogurt, and cheese—Gruyère from Switzerland
is a big winner, with 3 grams of leucine per 4 ounces of cheese.
That liquid that floats to the top of yogurt containers—don't
pour it down the drain. That liquid is nutritionally valuable
whey, which is an excellent source of protein—especially leucine. Just stir it back into the yogurt and enjoy, knowing that
it's making you stronger!

Importantly, you can consume 70 grams of protein a day—
including the required dose of leucine—*without* eating meat.
According to the Department of Agriculture, the average
American consumes 225 pounds of meat per year (not counting fish). That is about 10 ounces of steak, chicken, pork, lamb,
venison, elk, or guinea fowl every single day. Astounding! And
saddening. Yes, older Americans need more protein to ward
off declines in muscle mass, but this high level of meat consumption is not nutritionally necessary. Countries with better
health than ours consume significantly less meat—Denmark
at 160 pounds per year, Italy at 178, and Norway at 149.

The key nutrients of meat—essential amino acids like leucine, as well as vitamin B_{12}, iron, and other minerals—can all
be found in other foods. Again, eggs, dairy, yogurt, nuts, and

beans work. And there are reasons to avoid overconsumption of meat—it also loads you up with calories and saturated
fats with no beneficial fiber. Finally, high meat consumption is linked to heart disease, diabetes, cancer, and other
deadly conditions.

I like the taste of meat, and I think that it can have a place
in a healthy, balanced diet. Following the 80/20 rule, I call
myself an 80% vegetarian. I still eat meat but in limited
quantities. That translates to between 12 and 16 ounces a
week, or 40 to 50 pounds a year—less than a quarter of the
US average.

So if, like me, you choose to keep eating some meat, it is
important to be selective. Avoid processed meats like bacon,
salami, bologna, and other sandwich meats. They are bad. I
grew up on them for school lunches, but the more I learned,
the less good they tasted. They are associated with weight
gain, diabetes, heart disease, and many types of cancer.

But hey, I'm from Chicago, and a few times a year, I just
have to scarf a "Chicago dog"—or two or three—with all the
trimmings. And as kids, my brothers and I used to tag along
to deliver fine meats to Chicago area delis with my grand-
father, who was in the specialty foods business of importing
hams, bacon, and other foods from Denmark and distributing
specially-made beef products. So, the occasional corned beef
or pastrami on rye brings back fond memories and is something pleasurable to share with my mother. No reason to be
a purist but every reason not to be a pig. And the occasional
treat will not shave any minutes off your life, especially if you
enjoy it with someone you love.

Vegans who rely on plant proteins are at a disadvantage.
Without dairy or eggs, they really have to work hard on their
protein and especially leucine consumption. Most fruits and

vegetables are poor sources of protein, leucine, and vitamin B_{12} in particular. A few plant sources, including chickpeas and black, navy, and kidney beans, contain sufficient proteins and have a slightly higher concentration of essential amino acids such as leucine. But, compared with meat, you have to consume more calories for the same amount of protein. For instance, consuming the same amount of protein as in 4 ounces of meat would require about 2 cups of beans at roughly 1,000 calories. There are always trade-offs. Nuts are also good sources of protein and leucine. Per 4 ounces, pistachios have about 20 grams of protein and 4 grams of leucine. Blueberries, mushrooms, spinach, and beets have good amounts of vitamin B_{12}.

Protein powders can help supplement protein intake for vegans and vegetarians, but they are often highly processed and laced with sweeteners, real and artificial. Also, vegans who sprinkle on protein powders may inadvertently be doing themselves harm, as many protein powders have been shown to be contaminated with heavy metals like cadmium and lead. So, while vegans *can* get enough protein and leucine from whole foods, it takes mental focus and more planning—the opposite of not obsessing about wellness.

The fourth beneficial behavior involves **fiber**. If protein is today's dietary fad, fiber is likely to be tomorrow's. We all need fiber, but unlike our craving for protein, Americans generally do not get enough of it. There are two kinds of fiber. Insoluble fiber does not dissolve in water and passes through the body unchanged. Some insoluble fibers are called prebiotics and promote the growth of good gut bacteria. Soluble fibers do dissolve in water and form a gel-like substance that slows digestion and absorption of sugars and other nutrients but facilitates the bowels for regularity.

Fiber offers three main health advantages. First it slows uptake of sugars, blunting the unhealthy blood glucose surges and crashes. This explains why eating oranges and grape-fruits is better for you than drinking their juices—the fruit has way more fiber than the juice. Fiber also makes you feel full, thereby causing you to eat less. It also helps promote a good microbiome, heart and blood vessel health, and seems to reduce inflammation. A recent study of about 1,500 patients with stroke across 20 years found a stable linear correlation: as fiber intake goes up, stroke risk goes down at a consistent rate. In that same study, those in the group of highest fiber intake had 29% lower odds of stroke and 32% lower odds of dying from any cause compared with those in the group of lowest fiber intake.

Adults need approximately 30 to 35 grams of fiber a day. But according to a survey by the University of California, San Francisco, on average Americans get half the amount, 14 grams. In large part, that may be because Americans underconsume fruits and vegetables, the main source of fiber. The best foods to eat for fiber are fruits like raspberries, blackberries, pears, apples, and kiwi, vegetables like sweet potatoes, brussels sprouts, broccoli, and cauliflower, legumes like peas, lentils, chickpeas, and green beans, and nuts like pumpkin seeds and almonds. Finally, there are whole wheat products like bran and oats and whole grain breads and pas-tas. For those of you who don't find any of this appealing, pop-corn is a good source of fiber—but you have to eat a lot—3 cups for about 6 grams of fiber.

Let's be clear, eating food with fiber is a lot cheaper, tastier, and healthier than buying expensive prebiotic supplements. Don't waste your money. Eat the raspberries and broccoli.

You can be ahead of the next fad by eating your fiber now.

The fifth beneficial eating behavior is related to **fats**. For years, we were virtually brainwashed into thinking that eating fats will make you fat and that it is best to consume a low-fat diet. This has long since been proven wrong. It all depends on the kind of fats you eat. Fortunately, this is one of those food domains in which we have made great progress associated with weight gain.

There are really three types of fats to be aware of.

- *Trans fats*, which are made industrially when hydrogen is added to cooking oil. For food processing companies, trans fats are desirable because they turn liquid vegetable oils into a solid product that won't spoil and is cheap. Trans fats were essential to foods such as margarine and commercially baked goods, like those Milano cookies I gave my daughters. They are undesirable because they raise your risk of heart disease, diabetes, breast and colon cancer, and many other deadly maladies. Fortunately, artificial trans fats have been banned in the United States since 2018.
- *Saturated fats*, which are "saturated with hydrogen atoms" because they have only single bonds between carbon atoms—that's my chemistry training kicking in. They are solids at room temperature and typically found in butter, coconut oil, red meat, and cured meats like bacon. Saturated fats can also be found in healthier foods like eggs, milk, and cheese. Not all saturated fats are the same—some, like dairy saturated fats—seem to be neutral, if not beneficial. But there is medical consensus that too much saturated fat is not good for you. You can safely eat some saturated fat, but don't overdo it.
- *Unsaturated fats* are the other type of naturally occurring fats...and they are good for you. As someone trained in chemistry, I consider them as beneficial because some of the carbon atoms in the fatty acid chain have formed dou-

ble bonds, resulting in fewer hydrogen atoms. These long, double-bonded carbon chains are advantageous and even necessary in our bodies, playing a critical role in vitamin and nutrient absorption, blood clotting, and maintaining healthy cell membranes. As someone trained in medicine, I recognize the role that unsaturated fats play in reducing "bad" cholesterol and managing inflammation. Unsaturated fats are the fats found in olive oil and peanut oil, avocados, almonds, pecans, walnuts (and other nuts), flaxseed, and fish. Some are monounsaturated—they have one double carbon bond—and others are polyunsaturated—they have two or more double carbon bonds. Both are good for you. And those so-called fish oils are polyunsaturated and good for you, linked to reduced risk of heart disease and cancer. The key seems to be the omega-3s. Like essential amino acids, our bodies don't make them, so we only get them through eating. If you don't consume fish, you can get the omega-3s from flaxseeds, chia seeds, hemp hearts, walnuts, kidney beans, fish oil, or flaxseed supplements. Some health experts worry about omega-3 supplementation because they are associated with atrial fibrillation—where part of the heart beats irregularly and rapidly and can cause clots that are then pushed into the circulation. As one review put it, "The data from the 4 trials suggest, but do not prove, that there may be a dose related risk of AF [atrial fibrillation] with omega-3 fatty acid intake." Since the more you consume the greater the risk, if you are taking the supplement, the standard dose of 840 milligrams is the right amount, as it was not associated with any increased risk.

Contrary to some discussion of seed oils on the Internet, liquid plant oils are generally good for you. Extra-virgin olive oil is superior to all other oils for health benefits, but it is not cheap. If you can't afford to buy extra-virgin olive oil, you can still get plenty of health benefits from canola and sunflower oils. But stick to the organic, cold-pressed versions to ensure you don't get glyphosates, an herbicide used in the industrial cultivation of seed oil plants.

Overall, don't be afraid of fats. Embrace them, selectively! Focus on easy changes to incorporate more of the right types of heathy, unsaturated fats in your diet: swap bottled salad dressing for one that's made at home with olive oil, cook your food in unsaturated plant oils, and snack on sources of healthy fats like nuts.

Sixth on our list of positive behaviors is **unprocessed carbohydrates**. Carbohydrates are perceived as a food poison, largely due to their ubiquity in processed, packaged foods. And yes, the types of carbs in processed foods—think of cookies, chips, sugary cereals—are too easily digested and absorbed. They cause blood sugar levels to shoot way up—which causes a surge in insulin—before rapidly dropping back down. This is the definition of a food with a high glycemic index. The short-lived spike in blood sugar fails to keep you full and leads to overeating. Regularly consuming foods with a high glycemic index can lead to insulin resistance—where your body becomes less sensitive to insulin and unable to process sugar in your bloodstream. Studies have shown that diets rich in high glycemic foods increase the risk of diabetes, heart disease, and death.

But not all carbohydrates cause these problems—there are good "high-quality" carbohydrates. The key to distinguishing good from bad carbohydrates is the amount of fiber. Good carbohydrates include whole grain bread, oatmeal (but not the instant kind), fruits and vegetables, and beans, peas, and lentils.

One of America's favorite carbohydrates is the potato. On average, Americans eat over 125 pounds per year—about 6 ounces per day—of fried, baked, mashed, boiled, and roasted potatoes. Unfortunately, potatoes are not great for you. In one of my favorite dietary studies, researchers at Harvard looked at the dietary habits of doctors and nurses, identifying foods they ate and their impact on weight over the subsequent 20 years or so. The single worst food associated with weight gain? Potatoes in any form. (As I noted before, the best? Yogurt!)

Some disagree with my view on potatoes. The eminent scholar of nutrition Marion Nestle and my brother-in-law, who started a vegetarian restaurant chain in Boston, think I give potatoes a bad rap. They point out that the potato saved the Irish in the 19th century. That's true. If you are starving, I admit that potatoes can be nutritious enough to keep you alive. And some potato varieties, such as fingerlings, are healthier than others. But in 21st-century United States, where we tend to eat industrially produced potatoes, limiting potato consumption is probably wise.

The seventh healthful behavior on our list is to cut back on **salt**. I grew up with no added salt. Zero-added salt in any food. My father was a kidney doctor, and like most of the physicians of his era, he believed that salt causes high blood pressure and ultimately kidney damage. So my mom cooked with absolutely no added salt. I can't even recall our family having a saltshaker in our house. I grew up on the taste of real, home-cooked food. One consequence was that for most of my life, any dish that had just a few shakes of added salt was simply too salty for me.

Table 5: Best and Worst Foods for Weight Loss

	Food	Average Weight Gain or Loss (over a 4-year period)
WORST FOODS FOR WEIGHT GAIN	French fries	3.35 pounds
	Potato chips	1.69 pounds
	Sugar-sweetened beverages	1.0 pounds
	Red meat	0.95 pounds
	Processed meats (bologna)	0.93 pounds
BEST FOODS FOR WEIGHT LOSS	Fruits	0.49 pounds
	Nuts	0.57 pounds
	Yogurt	0.82 pounds

Source: Adapted from Dariush Mozaffarian et al., "Changes in Diet and Lifestyle and Long-Term Weight Gain in Women and Men," *New England Journal of Medicine* 364, no. 23 (June 2011): 2292–2404.

Almost all processed foods have way too much salt. Indeed, more than 70% of salt intake comes from processed foods. Canned soups, even those marketed as organic and healthy, are among the worst offenders. As one health website puts it, "The healthiest soups contain 360–600 milligrams of sodium per serving, but one cup of canned soup can contain 800 or more milligrams of sodium!" As the American Heart Association says, ideally, people would consume 1,500 milligrams of sodium per day. But acquiescing to the heavy salt palates of Americans, most recommendations are for a maximum of 2,300 milligrams per day. Still, that is just 1 teaspoon of salt for all the food you eat in a day. A single 1-cup serving of soup can be half of all the sodium you should consume. Another reason to avoid all that junk food—even organic junk food.

When you eat out, you can't control the salt content of your food—the chef or, at mass-market fast-food joints, the company does. Take McDonald's. Their classic, small Hamburger clocks in with 510 milligrams of salt, while a Double Quarter Pounder with Cheese has a whopping 1,360 milligrams of salt. Chick-fil-A says they take great care to make their menu nutritious. But their flagship Chick-fil-A Chicken sandwich has 1,460 milligrams of salt, and the deluxe version has 1,700 milligrams. The delicious Raising Cane's 4-finger Box Combo has 2,280 millgrams of salt.

Cutting back on salt has big health advantages. Recent research shows that for patients with high blood pressure—which is nearly half of all American adults—cutting salt intake to about 500 milligrams per day is an effective intervention. As the authors say, "The blood pressure–lowering effect of dietary sodium reduction was comparable with a commonly used first-line antihypertensive medication." Another recent study showed that not using added salt also reduced the risk of developing chronic kidney disease. People "who said they always added extra salt to their food had an 11% higher risk for developing chronic kidney disease compared with those who never or only rarely added salt."

Conclusion: My mom and dad were right. Zero-added salt is best. But most people are not going to get there, and we shouldn't waste our willpower trying. We can make progress by reducing the processed foods we eat and reducing how often we eat out, especially at fast-food restaurants. And we can shake a little less into our home-cooked meals—just use *one* pinch of the salt rather than two. It will take a few months for your taste buds to recalibrate, but cutting back on the sodium is much better and cheaper than taking two or three blood pressure drugs or ending up on dialysis because of kidney failure.

The eighth dietary recommendation concerns **alcohol**. I won't scold or scare anyone into being a teetotaler. But alcohol consumption may be one of the most studied topics in nutrition. For many years, alcohol was viewed positively, and red wine in particular was thought to be healthy because of antioxidants such as resveratrol. But recent research has placed alcohol back in the penalty box.

Alcohol consumption beyond half or one drink a day is definitely not healthy, and it increases the risk of developing a wide range of diseases. For instance, along with asbestos, smoking, and UV radiation, alcohol has been classified as a "group 1 carcinogen," the highest risk category for cancers. Substances in this group are *known* to cause cancer in humans. Alcohol in particular has been linked to colon, breast, throat, esophagus, and liver cancers. About 4% of all cancers are attributed to alcohol. Beyond cancer, alcohol also causes liver cirrhosis. It also increases the risk of hypertension. A small exception may be people at risk for heart disease, particularly middle-aged men, for whom moderate consumption of alcohol is associated with lower risk of mortality. But for the general population, alcohol is bad for your body.

Alcohol is also bad for brain function. Consuming 2 or more alcoholic drinks a day (14 per week) is associated with brain atrophy and dementia. Indeed, a study of nearly 314,000 people in Great Britain found that there is a linear relationship between alcohol intake and dementia—the more you drink, the greater the risk. Or as the researchers concluded: "Our findings suggested that there was no safe level of alcohol consumption for dementia."

Overall, this suggests that between zero and 1 drink per

day is the limit before you tip into anti-wellness, unless you happen to be a middle-aged man for whom moderate alcohol use protects against heart disease. So don't consume alcohol every day, and try to keep it to one drink when you decide to partake. This may be a tough ask, but it is what the data suggest. Maybe most importantly, drinking should be with other people, not alone, to ensure there is the compensating health benefit from the sociability.

The penultimate recommendation is about eating **organic**. Let's be honest. The main barrier to eating organic is money. If organic food were priced the same as nonorganic food and readily available, most people would surely choose to eat organic. But this is not because organic food is more nutritious than nonorganic food. As some experts claim: "There isn't a concrete study that proves organic foods lead to healthier children." This cautious phrasing is important. As the saying goes, the absence of evidence does not mean there is evidence of absence.

Although it may be true that organic and nonorganic foods contain the same nutrients, those pesticides, hormones, and other additives in and on nonorganic foods cannot be good for you. Children who don't eat organic consume higher levels of pesticides. Exposure to pesticides is linked to attention-deficit/hyperactivity disorder (ADHD), autism, reduced cognitive skills like memory, and especially in later life, Parkinson's disease and cancer. Pesticides are designed to kill bugs. When they get into our gut, they don't suddenly stop killing bugs. As researchers have written, "Low-level chronic dietary exposure to pesticides can affect the human gut microbiota." I have often wondered whether the use of pesticides to treat nonorganic wheat has some role in the 7.5% annual increase in celiac disease over the last 50 years. As scientists always say, we need more research.

Finally, as the food critic and my friend Corby Kummer notes, we are not only eating for ourselves. What we eat affects others. The pesticides, hormones, and chemicals mixed into nonorganic foods are either neutral or bad for you in low doses. But the frequent high doses of pesticides are dangerous to the agriculture workers and to the groundwater. So if you can afford it, why take the risk?

I now come to the last, and in my view, the most important dietary recommendation. What to do about **dessert**? As a child, my family would take car trips from Chicago to Colorado, Utah, South Dakota, Montana, California, and all the states in between. One of my main memories of these trips is that my brothers and I would order cherry pie every opportunity we could. Today, I love to bake and do so regularly. I am especially proud of my apple crisps, banana cake, and cheesecake (a recipe from my mother). Indeed, I like baking so much that I recently received a holiday gift for a 4-hour pie crust class at King Arthur's Baking Company in Vermont. I learned a ton, including how to flute the crust.

I also love chocolate and even make the "Zeke Bar," a single-origin bean-to-bar chocolate with Askinosie Chocolate, in Springfield, Missouri. This journey began many years ago when I was the master of ceremonies (MC) at the Good Food Awards, an event that recognizes food makers across the United States for their expertly crafted beers, ciders, and coffees as well as oils, mustards, honeys, cheese, preserves, and . . . chocolate. That year, Shawn Askinosie, one of the original single-origin bean-to-bar makers in the United States, was a winner. We began talking about chocolate, and I asked if I could make a bar with him. He said he had received hundreds of such requests, and no one ever persisted enough to make a bar. But I pestered and pestered and pestered. In part, I was driven by my commitment to do one totally new thing that I had never done before every year. Finally, Shawn and I went to Madagascar to get beans, helped to harvest and process them, and imported them to his factory. Then I worked with the team for a week straight, roasting, winnowing, grinding, conching, plating, and tempering to produce about 2,500 bars. The majority of the proceeds go to Chocolate University, Shawn's charity, to take underprivileged students from Springfield to Tanzania to work with the cocoa farmers and their families. I have now gone back to Springfield many times to make multiple bars.

This love of desserts and chocolate poses a conundrum for me—health versus passion. So here are my recommendations. Consider dessert a special occasion, something you do episodically—a couple of times a week, and in small portions. You should avoid having dessert every night, especially the cake and cookie kind with lots of sugar, refined flours, and saturated fats. Great choices for more frequent "sweet treats" include fresh fruit—grapes, apples, strawberries, clementines, mangos, peaches, apricots, watermelon on those hot summer days—and nuts, like pistachios. You can also make cheese a dessert.

I have been told that my chocolate obsession is not bad. Dark chocolate of over 70% cocoa, especially with nuts, can be an excellent, healthy dessert. A few squares and you are in heaven. And, I find the good thing about chocolate dessert is that it's hard to overeat. Too much makes you feel sick. Make the indulgence worth it with good-quality dark chocolate. Milk chocolate appeals to many people, but has less antioxidant-rich cocoa solids and more sugar, which is again training you to eat sweet things.

In addition to Askinosie, my favorite chocolate makers are Goodnow Farms, Dick Taylor, Soma from Canada, and Fjåk from Norway. But even easy-to-find producers like Lindt are a relatively healthy, delicious, and cheap alternative.

Finally, there is ice cream. It would seem to be a nutritional disaster—especially those delectable premium brands. They are high in calories, saturated (bad) fat, cholesterol, and sugar—the epitome of junk food. Argh!!

Or so we may think. But a recent article in *The Atlantic* explored whether ice cream might not only *not* be bad, but might even offer health benefits. The article noted that for 20 years the health benefits of ice cream have been well known among nutrition scientists, but because this insight defied traditional wisdom, it has not been widely publicized. (Defenders argue it was included in academic papers, just not highlighted or emphasized. Skeptics ask who funded the studies and how much dairy money went to the researchers.)

Researchers found that ice cream improves people's health and is associated with weight loss and reduced risk of diabetes and heart disease. This was the research conclusion despite "analyzing the hell out of the data" to be certain that the association was a real observation, not an artifact. An even more interesting finding is that "among diabetics, eating half a cup of ice cream a day was associated with a lower risk of heart problems." Yes, you read it right, ice cream *lowered* the risk of heart problems. Indeed, "ice cream was associated for overweight people with dramatically reduced odds of developing insulin-resistance syndrome."

The reasons are unclear. One theory is that there is something healthy about the fat globules in dairy. Remember, dairy is actually associated with a lower risk of diabetes. For those of us trying to eat well, we have a truly life-changing result: Ice cream is healthy—or at least not unhealthy! No longer a guilty pleasure. Break out a scoop of premium rocky road. But don't overdo it—ice cream still has plenty of calories and sugar—but make that premium stuff a guilt-free treat *occasionally*.

But you also need to be careful about other ingredients, avoiding those with artificial emulsifiers like polysorbate 80. This emulsifier is added to adjust the consistency of the scoops. But polysorbate 80 is very unhealthy for the same reason ultra-processed foods are. It reduces the microbiome diversity, triggers inflammation, and damages the gut's lining. So enjoy ice cream but avoid those with emulsifiers.

If you can do all this—stop the sodas and cut down on the snacks, reduce the ultra-processed foods to say 20% of calories, eat more fermented foods, dairy, unprocessed carbohydrates, and unsaturated fats, with less meat and salt, and stick to good desserts occasionally—you are almost all the way to health and wellness.

I admit that is a lot of change. And too much for most of us to do. Certainly too much to do all at once. But it is the roadmap for eating well. And I hope it is clear. Just start at the top—stopping sodas and reducing snacks—and work your way down the list, a little at a time. See how far you can go without going crazy. Don't obsess. Do what you can, but just make it a habit that fits into your life. Just don't get overwhelmed, do nothing, and continue bad eating habits.

But it's not just what you eat or don't eat; it's also how you eat that matters.

Every year I hire assistants to help me with my classes and conduct health policy or bioethics research. Typically, they are sharp, dedicated young adults a few years out of college, and they care deeply about health issues. One year, I saw them going out every day to buy lunch. I was surprised by how much they were spending on lunches because when I was their age, working at a lab in Oxford, I was so broke I was eating just two meals a day . . . and neither was bought. But more importantly, I was totally distraught about their nutrition.

When we discussed it, I learned that they had no idea how to cook. Their parents never taught them how to make an omelet, much less roast a chicken or whip up a lentil soup. And long ago, home economics was removed from high school curricula. I gave them my favorite roast chicken recipe, but it was a challenge to make. Used to eating out every day, they had no roasting pan or any of the usual ingredients—mustard, olive oil, root vegetables. When I encouraged them to cook more at home and slowly accrue the necessary equipment, one of them texted me a picture of one of Penn's Olympic swimmers walking on campus eating out of a Raising Cane's chicken container. It was accompanied by the comment, "We can sleep soundly now that we know we eat like an Olympian."

An Olympian or not, it is nearly impossible to eat well if you don't cook for yourself. Living on a steady diet of processed foods or fast foods is assuredly anti-wellness. It is not impossible to eat well on take-out food, but it takes real work—and attention to portion size and the details of nutritional content. Not only will it be onerous to constantly ask for nutritional information and ingredients, but eating out is both more expensive and, for most people, less fulfilling than cooking at home. Unfortunately, most people growing up in the last 40 years have little experience with the stove and pots and pans. Changing this habit can make a huge difference to your overall health and well-being.

For those who don't know how to cook but want to, a good strategy is to try one new recipe every week. Out of 21 meals a week, make one new soup, overnight oats, quiche, pasta, Chicken Marbella, fish, taco spread, or Middle Eastern meal. At the end of just one year, you will have mastered 52 different dishes and significantly improved your nutritional intake. And you'll have stretched your brain and spiced up your life.

Having learned to cook, you can throw a dinner party to show off your new skills. Robert Putnam, the author of *Bowling Alone*, wrote about the decline of civic engagement and social connection in the United States. An even bigger trend— and problem—is eating alone. Meals are not just for nutrients. They are inextricably linked with friendship by facilitating social interactions. The French word *copain* (friend), the Italian word *compagno* (mate), and the English word "companion" all come from the Latin words *cum* and *pānis*, literally "with-bread." The Chinese term for companion/partner, 伙 伴, stems from a similar term (火伴) that literally translates to "fire mate," a reference to sharing meals over a campfire.

It is shocking how frequently people eat alone. A survey in England done by Robin Dunbar, the expert in friendship, found that "a third of weekday evening meals are eaten in isolation, and the average adult eats 10 meals out of 21 alone every week ... 69% of those questioned had never shared a meal with any of their neighbors, while a fifth of people said it had been more than 6 months since they had shared a meal with their parents." More recently, in 2023, 25% of Americans reported eating *all of their meals alone*. That's an increase of 53% since 2003. This is a problem.

Eating together leads to all sorts of positives. People who eat with other people, especially at dinner, "feel happier and are more satisfied with life, are more trusting of others, are more engaged with their local communities, and have more friends they can depend on for support." Conversely, eating alone is associated with worse dietary habits, such as eating fewer vegetables and eating more prepared and junk food, and greatly contributes to loneliness. Loneliness is deadly, and even if it doesn't kill you, it makes the time you have on earth a lot worse. One of the easiest ways to be with people is to invite them over for a meal you cooked. You can even regale them on how you learned the recipe and what making the meal taught you. The benefits are less about the food itself—although it will almost inevitably be healthier than a take-out or store-bought meal—and more about sharing time together.

Eating as a family is hugely beneficial for children. When I was raising my children, we ate both breakfast and dinner together—14 meals a week. At breakfast, we would talk about what would be happening that day—any big events in school, like a test or performance, who would be picking them up, the planned after-school activities, and anything special that was happening for mom or dad. At dinner, we would review what happened during the day, and as the children grew up, we discussed the news of the day. We used meals as an opportunity to spend intentional time together, even during busy periods of our lives.

The distinguished epidemiologist and expert on health behavior Karen Glanz has reviewed the literature and documented the benefits of eating as a family. These shared family meals are associated with children consuming more fruits, vegetables, and healthful nutrients. Other studies link shared meals with positive health and psychosocial outcomes in youth, including less obesity, decreased risk for eating disorders, and improved academic achievement. Another literature review corroborates these results, finding that more frequent family meals are associated with fewer eating disorders, less alcohol or substance abuse, as well as less "violent behavior . . . and feelings of depression or thoughts of suicide in adolescents." It also improves school performance and self-esteem. These studies are far from perfect, and the scientist in me will emphasize that these studies do not show eating together *causes* these health and social benefits. They are associated. My upshot is that there is no downside to family meals and probably many benefits. So, one way you can show you care about your children's long-term health is to eat with them.

When your children are old enough, you can also teach them to cook. Whenever I am with my grandchildren, we make granola together. They love measuring out the oats and nuts, mixing them with oil and maple syrup, and smelling the cinnamon or nutmeg or cardamom. It also teaches them delayed gratification, as they have to wait for the granola to cook and then cool before tasting.

Finally, eating together means being present in mind, not just in body. When I was growing up, my mother prohibited answering the telephone during dinner. That was in the era of landlines and no social media. Today, her restriction means no cell phones or social media. My modification of my mom's rule is to have no phones at the table, and wherever they are, the ringer is turned off. Concentrate on having a conversation with your eating companions and mastering the fine art of asking questions, listening, and learning.

Besides learning to cook and eating with other people, the last "how" to eat involves timing and the growing question of intermittent fasting. You would think determining when we should eat would be simple. Morning, noon, and night. It turns out that like the microbiome, this is one of those topics that had long been ignored but may be important. A whole new scientific field developed over the last 10 to 15 years—*chrononutrition*.

One fundamental lesson of this new science is that when during the day we eat *does* seem to matter to health. This is likely because our daily eating time "is a dominant synchronizer of the circadian" cycle in many of our organs. What do we know about when to eat?

First, eat breakfast. Omitting breakfast is associated with obesity, heart disease, and diabetes. That's right, *not* eating breakfast is associated with problems we usually think are related to overeating. Also, breakfast should be your big meal, not a power bar snack or carbohydrate or sugar-filled doughnut or croissant. Think eggs and yogurt with fruit and nuts—high in protein, good fats, and fiber and low in sugar. Compared with eating breakfast late in the morning, defined as after 9 a.m., eating breakfast early, before 8 a.m., seems to reduce the risk of heart disease. Second, avoid late-night snacking because it leads to obesity, heart disease, and, at least in women, metabolic syndrome, which is like prediabetes. For reducing the risk of heart disease, eating dinner before 8 p.m. seems better than eating after 8 p.m. and especially after 9 p.m. Finally, there is evidence that longer periods of time between dinner and breakfast the next morning can reduce the risk of stroke.

This brings us to the question of intermittent fasting. I think the idea of the wellness benefits from intermittent fasting first arose because of experiments demonstrating that restricted caloric intake in worms, fish, and mice extended average and maximal lifespans. While these findings were first reported over 70 years ago, they have more recently spurred research on the wellness and longevity effects of both the timing of meals and the periods of fasting. These studies show that consuming fewer calories leads to less obesity, diabetes, heart disease, and cancer. When the body is fasting, cells activate special pathways that favor maintenance and repair, specifically inhibiting protein synthesis and stimulating the breaking down of defective cells and recycling of proteins and other molecules. These pathways also trigger DNA repair, lessening of inflammation, and increasing the number and size of the energy-producing mitochondria in cells. All of these changes promote cellular resilience and cell survival and thus improve health. Today, the research is moving from worms and mice to people. Some data suggest that diabetics who crammed all their eating into 8 hours—breakfast at 8 a.m. and dinner no later than 4 p.m., for instance—and thus had 16 hours between dinner and subsequent breakfast—could lose weight and in some cases reverse their diabetes. This worked for eating in a 10-hour interval too, but if the time between breakfast and dinner expanded to 12 hours or longer, the health benefits evaporated.

Despite some promising studies, it is hard to be definitive about intermittent fasting. Scientists haven't found enough compelling data to endorse it for a wide population, but there are many glimmers of potential benefit. In 2019, two researchers published a review of intermittent fasting in *The New England Journal of Medicine* touting its benefits—noting that some data suggest that fasting "slows or reverses aging and disease processes." Subsequently, other researchers have cast doubt on some of the claims for intermittent fasting. In part this is because there are so many different ways to define fasting, which influences the outcomes. Should you fast for 24 hours once a week, or 16 hours a day, or define fasting as eating just 500 calories a day? The goal could be weight loss, lower risk of heart disease and cancer, or living longer. Long-term observational population studies also tend to have a problem: People who engage in intermittent fasting also follow other healthy habits, confounding definitive conclusions. On the flip side, randomized trials tend to be short term—weeks to months—because few researchers can wait years until publishing their results. And yet wellness and longevity are about the long-term benefits of behaviors.

What to do? For the vast majority of people, intermittent fasting may have a few benefits and no downsides. If you are going to try intermittent fasting, remember that the key biological effects begin after about 12 hours, when the body uses up its glucose stores and begins using fatty acids for energy. This reaches a maximum at 24 hours. Thus, you have to fast longer than 12 hours to see the benefits. That kind of fasting almost certainly will lead to some weight loss. I've tried it, and the result was losing about 5 to 8 pounds over 4 months.

The biggest challenge is sticking with it. Most people I know find the hunger, irritability, and inability to concentrate from fasting quite problematic. For me, the biggest problem is that I get very cold after about 18 hours. If you want to do intermittent fasting, you have to recognize the triggers. I get hungry for a 1-hour stretch after about 18 hours of fasting. So I make sure during that time to avoid the kitchen or walking by food stores and restaurants. Instead, I plan to drink (water and tea!) during that time. Like every habit, however, fasting becomes easier the more you do it, and after a couple of months, these feelings dissipate.

My personal routine is fasting for 24 hours one day a week. I try to go from breakfast to breakfast, so the last 8 hours are while I am asleep with no important meetings or decisions to make. Toward the later part of the night of a fast day, 15 to 18 or so hours into the fast, when the body switches to fatty acids as its energy source, I begin to get cold, but this actually helps me sleep more soundly.

But let's be clear, intermittent fasting is absolutely not *necessary* for wellness or longevity. If you are just starting a wellness routine, it is much better to expend your limited willpower on integrating other behaviors into your routine— such as quitting soda and keeping up with friends and family. But for anyone looking to experiment with a new wellness behavior, intermittent fasting can complement the benefits of otherwise eating well.

———

The last topic is maybe the most argued about: **supplements**. As many as 75% of adult Americans take supplements, often multiple. Unfortunately, thanks to Senator Orrin Hatch of Utah—where many supplement producers are located—the FDA lost its authority to regulate supplements in 1994, sending us back to the days of quackery and snake oil.

Some supplements are downright dangerous. Vitamins A and E increase cancer risks. So, too, does beta-carotene a precursor to vitamin A. And some supplements have been shown to contain contaminants and toxins such as heavy metals, pesticides, dioxins, or fungi.

Some supplements are beneficial—but usually only for certain populations. Folate is good for women considering pregnancy. Folate reduces neural tube defects in babies—think spina bifida. Because of this, folate is added to grains—like flour, bread, pasta, and rice. Still, for women of childbearing age, it is worth taking supplements. (Many if not most pregnant women will also need iron, vitamin D, and vitamin B_{12}.) And for vegetarians, vegans, and older people whose stomachs don't make enough acid, vitamin B_{12} supplementation is very important.

For most of the other supplements, the evidence is not definitive. Advice about vitamin D has become a morass of misunderstanding. Many people get tests for vitamin D levels unnecessarily. There is huge controversy over what constitutes vitamin D deficiency because the standards for sufficiency and deficiency are all over the place. Regardless, the majority of people do get enough vitamin D. It is best captured from about 15 to 30 minutes a day in the sun—without sunscreen. And we store about a 10- to 12-week supply of vitamin D in our liver. Think about how people in the upper reaches of Canada and Norway and Sweden survive when not getting enough sunshine during the dark northern winters. They also eat fatty fish containing plenty of vitamin D. If you are worried, getting outside and in nature is the cheapest and psychologically superior way to get more vitamin D. If you can't for some reason, a 1,000 IU vitamin D supplement will do it. It is also important to remember that breastfed babies might need some vitamin D supplements.

There are also fish oil and flaxseed oil supplements that offer omega-3 fatty acids. These fatty acids are beneficial, stimulating hair and skin growth, protecting against cardio-vascular disease, and reducing inflammation. But, as I mentioned, they also have a downside risk of atrial fibrillation. So, take no more than 1 gram a day. There are other ways of getting these fatty acids—like eating fish or nuts. But for those people who don't get enough, supplements may not hurt.

Multivitamins are big business in the United States. Americans spend about $12 billion on multivitamins, and over 70% of seniors take one. But multivitamins are not beneficial. They do not reduce heart disease or cancer or dementia. The Physicians' Health Study II randomized 14,641 male doctors to either a multivitamin or a placebo and followed them for over 11 years. The result: No benefit in terms of heart disease. The vitamins might have reduced the total number of cancers by 1 for every 1,000 people taking them. There was no slowing of cognitive decline either. Data from a meta-analysis of multiple studies that followed people for up to 27 years showed that multivitamins, vitamin E, and other supplements don't help with longevity or heart disease or cancer. As a group of Johns Hopkins researchers who reviewed the literature put it: "Enough is Enough: Stop Wasting Money on Vitamin and Mineral Supplements."

Then there are plenty of supplements, such as taurine or

NADH, that people choose to take based on some rationale from animal studies or possibly a few small human studies. For instance, a few years ago, some reputable medical organizations proclaimed taurine supplements might be the "elixir of life" because of studies in mice. But more recent studies of taurine from the National Institutes of Health suggest that taurine is important for health, but taurine supplments are not. As the researchers stated: "On the basis of these findings, we conclude that low circulating taurine concentrations are unlikely to serve as a good biomarker of aging." The upshot is that the data on most of these supplments are all over the place and weak. Ask reputable physicians and almost all will retort, "There are no definitive data, more research is needed." Nevertheless, many people believe that if it is not going to do harm, the only downside is expensive urine.

My bottom line on supplements: Folate and iron for women of childbearing age. Vitamin B_{12} for vegetarians, vegans, and the elderly. Vitamin D for those who don't get 15 minutes of sunlight a day. The rest is at your discretion but probably a waste of money.

The conclusions about eating well are pretty simple:

- Reduce sodas and other sugary drinks to an absolute minimum—zero is best but once a week is okay. Diet drinks are no better. Drink water, tea, or coffee instead.
- Limit cookies, doughnuts, and other packaged snacks. Again, zero is best but having them once a week or so is not the end of the world. Substitute fruit and nuts as much as possible for daily snacks.
- Reduce ultra-processed junk foods to about 20% of calories per day.

- Eat fermented foods like yogurt and kimchi.
- Eat dairy products.
- Ensure that you get enough protein, particularly leucine.
- Avoid unprocessed carbohydrates and limit saturated fats, especially from meats.
- Reduce meat intake to a pound a week, and eliminate processed meats except for special occasions.
- Consume less salt by cooking at home.
- If you eat desserts, make them occasional.

Remember, it is also important not to be extreme. You can have pastries, a hot dog, a can of soda, and or a piece of cake. Just make it occasional, not routine, and in small quantities. And once you establish and maintain good eating habits, stop obsessing about it and focus on the important things in life, like cooking and enjoying a meal with friends.

5

Move It!

Exercising Well and Regularly

My father never "exercised." He did not regularly run, play soccer, ride a bicycle, swim laps, do yoga, or lift weights. Indeed, the cheapskate in him would have considered a gym membership a waste of money. But he was forever known as Speedy. He walked, and walked fast. Every morning my father would go to three or four hospitals, examine a newborn baby, walk to the mother's room to give his special "well baby talk," and then zip to the next baby or child under his care. He was called Speedy because before you knew it, he was off to the next patient. As children, we would go on hospital rounds with him on weekends. And I vividly remember literally running with the nurses behind him trying to keep up.

His favorite vacations were at national parks. We would spend the nights camping, and the days hiking up and down the trails. Speedy was always in front, and we were always scrambling behind until we became teenagers and could run ahead.

He and my mother were fantastic dancers. At weddings, bar and bat mitzvahs, and other celebrations, they would dance enthusiastically for hours—often while other couples just watched.

All his life, my father was skinny and fast—that is, until his 70s when something happened in his neck. As a "good" doctor, he was terribly averse to medical care and refused to see a surgeon. He cut down on all his walking and no longer walked fast. The consequences were terrible: he gained weight, developed type 2 diabetes, and eventually had a heart attack—which, again, as a good doctor, he dismissed for three weeks as acid indigestion. Eventually, he cut out sugar and by sheer dietary control got off his diabetes medications with normal blood sugar. But he never got back to being Speedy.

I guess being speedy is genetic or otherwise inherited. Besides my father, no one has ever told me or my brothers that we needed to walk faster. My daughters recall similar memories of how, as children, they had to chase behind me when we walked to the bookstore or down the aisles at the grocery store. The familial pattern continues—my youngest daughter was the zippiest walker at her college, with friends trotting beside her to class.

Speed walking is aerobic exercise—good for the heart—and even better because it doesn't require a gym membership or special equipment. Indeed, my father's preferred exercise is the kind found in the Blue Zones, where centenarians don't necessarily run, swim laps, or lift weights but instead walk, hike, and garden. Even if you don't formally "exercise," you can certainly get enough physical activity to raise your heart rate and keep yourself healthy, provided you do it regularly. And as my father showed, if you stop being physically active, you lose fitness and become susceptible to serious and life-threatening chronic illnesses. Exercise is a magical path to wellness and longevity. Plus, if you do it right, it is not arduous or burdensome but fun and fulfilling.

The problem is that Americans are not getting enough exercise. An assessment of nearly 32,000 Americans in the National Health Interview Survey found that only a meager 28% of Americans exercise enough. That means that 72% of Americans get too little physical activity and are shortchanging their lives. Perhaps this is because 82% of Americans prefer sedentary leisure activities—watching movies and TV shows, playing video games, cheering for their favorite sports team, and the like. On average, American adults spend nearly 10 hours a day sitting. The real secret of exercise is simple. You don't have to be an Olympian to reap the benefits of movement. Be like Speedy, and just do some.

While a large majority of Americans fail to get sufficient exercise, that's not even the worst of it. The same survey showed that 25% of individuals are couch potatoes—that is, they are completely or almost completely physically inactive. Being a couch potato is dangerous. You may remember that I think potatoes are nutritionally lacking. It's no surprise that being a couch potato is the human equivalent—it epitomizes an anti-wellness and anti-longevity lifestyle.

The crazy thing is that we have known the harm of physical inactivity since at least 1953, when British researchers studied the health differences between London bus drivers and bus conductors. Drivers remained seated at the wheel all day, while conductors roamed the bus, traversing the stairs of London's renowned double-deckers to collect fares. Sedentary drivers were significantly more prone to experiencing heart attacks than were the physically active conductors and were *nearly twice as likely to die of heart disease.* This finding holds true today, as "incidence of coronary heart-disease is lower in the [physically active] postmen than in the sedentary" government workers, with mortality approximately halved in postmen as compared to their inactive counterparts.

Regular physical activity—not just the one-off trip to the gym, but routine, habitual, instinctive movement—is essential for wellness. It reduces the risk of the big killers: heart disease, cancer, stroke, diabetes, high blood pressure, dementia, and even infectious diseases. It can also positively affect your mental health, reducing depression and anxiety. Even more, exercise can help people with chronic illnesses, such as diabetes, manage their disease and avoid exacerbations that can compromise quality of life.

According to the World Health Organization, people who are "insufficiently active have a 20% to 30% increased risk of death compared to people who are sufficiently active." A meta-analysis covering over 30 million participants found that as many as 1 in 10 premature deaths could be avoided if everyone were to get half the recommended 150 minutes per week of physical activity. What does this mean for the average person? A study in Taiwan followed over 400,000 men and women between 1996 and 2008. Exercising as little as 15 minutes per day (over 90 minutes per week) was associated with an extra 3 years of life. Yes, 3 years! And each additional 15 minutes of daily exercise added just under 1 additional year.

But the effects are not limited to increasing lifespan and decreasing incidence of disease. Exercise may also enhance brain function. In one study, researchers enrolled 160 older individuals who were largely sedentary and beginning to have cognitive problems—such as difficulty with memory and concentration or challenges with executive functions like decision-making—but did not meet the criteria of dementia. Baseline cognitive tests demonstrated that participants had an average "mental" age of a 93-year-old, approximately 28 years older than their chronological age. They were given either 6 months of education on enhancing brain function or a program involving moderate exercise for 45 minutes 3 times a week, coupled with a DASH diet (similar to the guidelines I recommended in the previous chapter). The exercise and diet group had significant improvement in their executive functioning. One year follow-up cognitive testing showed that this regimen improved executive function by almost 8 years.

Exercise also has the side benefit of improving other essential elements of wellness: sleep, social relationships, and stress. Exercise is proven to improve sleep duration and quality, even for those with insomnia or other sleep difficulties. It can also have a positive impact on social relationships, as a meaningful activity to do with another person. Perhaps in part because of these many positive associations, exercise is also recommended for reducing stress. As the Mayo Clinic says: "Virtually any form of exercise, from aerobics to yoga, can act as a stress reliever. If you're not an athlete or even if you're out of shape, you can still make a little exercise go a long way toward stress management."

If you are at all interested in wellness and living a healthy life—and you must be, because you bought this book—stop procrastinating. Just get off your ass and move around. Don't spend your leisure time sitting around in front of a screen doomscrolling or online shopping. The biggest gains in reducing the risk of death are found in people who go from no activity to doing some moderate exercise. Transitioning from being horizontal to walking, progressing to jogging or hiking up hills, then to running or biking offers the biggest potential improvement in your wellness and longevity. Add some amount of exercise to your routine.

Why does exercise have such an impact on health and wellness? What happens to your body when you work out? Exercise demands more oxygen throughout the body, forcing the heart to pump faster and eject larger volumes of blood every time it squeezes. This strengthens the heart muscle, but more importantly, it spawns an increase in blood vessel formation and diameter in the heart and musculature. The increase in the heart's blood vessels improves blood flow to the heart, which is critical for its function. If there is blockage in one vessel, these other blood vessels create what cardiologists call "collateral flow" around the blockage, which can ensure continued delivery of blood to all the heart tissue. This collateral flow also reduces the long-term chances of having and dying from a heart attack. Sustained exercise also improves cholesterol, increasing the "good" (HDL) cholesterol and lowering the bad (LDL) cholesterol and triglycerides. This, too, reduces the risk of heart attacks.

On a cellular level, endurance exercise also increases the number and functional efficiency of mitochondria in the muscle—the power plant of cells that produce cellular energy (ATP). It increases the uptake of glucose and fatty acids, ultimately creating more energy for muscle contraction. Exercise also increases the sensitivity of cells to insulin, meaning they extract more glucose from the blood, leading to improved blood sugar control.

Finally, exercise places stress on your muscles, causing microtears. This minute damage is good for you. After exercise, the body repairs this damage and produces stronger muscles. A similar idea goes for bones, for which exercise and weight-bearing stress serve as mechanical cues for strength-

ening them. Exercise and other weight-bearing activities—
that is, not being sedentary—also increase the mineral density
of our bones. And bone density reduces the risk of fractures. A
perfect example are astronauts who lose bone density because
they lack weight-bearing activities in the zero gravity of
space. That is why the International Space Station is outfitted
with exercise equipment.

When someone recommends "exercise," your mind probably narrows in on running, swimming, rowing, biking, and
the like. That is aerobic exercise, which primarily impacts
and improves your cardiovascular health. But you need to
think bigger. There are two other types of essential exercise:
strength training and balance and flexibility training. It's
important to do all three kinds of exercise at every stage of life.

Aerobic exercise makes your heart, lungs, and circulatory
system work harder to deliver more oxygen to your muscles,
brain, and other organs. Over time, your muscles and organs
become more efficient and resistant to failure. The intensity
of aerobic exercise is determined by how much your heart
rate increases relative to your maximum heart rate. Your
maximum heart rate is age related and is crudely approxi-
mated by the simple formula 220 minus your age. If you are
60, your maximum heart rate is 160 beats per minute (220
minus 60). *Moderate* activity must increase your heart rate to
between 50% and 70% of your maximum heart rate. Thus, for
a 60-year-old, moderate activity is a heart rate of between 80
and 112. You should still be able to hold a conversation, though
you may choose your words more carefully. *Vigorous* activity requires getting your heart rate to between 70% and 85%
of your maximum heart rate. So vigorous activity and beyond
is anything that gets a 60-year-old's heart rate over 112 beats
per minute. With more physical activity, the body becomes

more fit, and these ranges should shift to become higher over time. You won't know your exact heart rate unless you have a wearable device, and I'm not trying to convince you to get one. Except for some valid clinical reason, you don't need to and shouldn't worry about tracking your heart rate. Instead, just use Table 6 and use the talk test: During moderate-intensity activities, you should be able to talk but not sing. During vigorous-intensity activities, you should not be able to say more than a few words without needing to pause for a breath. Table 6 shows a few activities in each category.

Table 6. Different Kinds of Aerobic Activity

Moderate Exercise 50–70% of Maximum Heart Rate	Vigorous Exercise 70–85% of Maximum Heart Rate
Brisk walking (15–20-minute miles)	Jogging or running (faster than 10-minute miles)
Hiking with little or no elevation change	Hiking up and down hills
Slow bicycling (10–12 miles per hour)	Moderate to intense bicycling (over 14 miles per hour)
Volleyball	Basketball, swimming laps, playing soccer, tennis, ice hockey
Housework and mowing the lawn	Jumping rope
	Ballroom dancing

Source: "Target Heart Rates Chart," American Heart Association, last modified August 12, 2024, accessed March 25, 2025.

Some experts and athletes use a more granular scale to categorize aerobic exercise into 5 or 6 different zones of intensity. Muscles and cells respond differently at each zone, using different types of energy and creating different waste products. Some researchers have postulated that

Zone 2—moderate-intensity endurance training—is optimal for developing mitochondria, reducing fat, and ultimately losing weight. Given its alignment with most fitness goals, Zone 2 training has become a sensation on social media, some calling it "the biggest thing in fitness."

But is Zone 2 training really the secret to optimizing your exercise routine? Most likely not. Researchers have tested the big claims of Zone 2 enthusiasts by, if you can believe it, repeatedly biopsying muscles from people exercising and tracking changes in their mitochondria. Compared with other types of exercise, such as high-intensity interval training and sprint interval training, Zone 2 endurance training actually produced less mitochondrial growth. In fact, "per total hour of exercise, SIT [sprint interval training] was ~3.9 times more efficient than ET [endurance or Zone 2 training], while HIT [high-intensity interval training] was ~1.7 times more efficient than ET" at increasing mitochondrial content in muscles. Seems like advocates of Zone 2 are in the twilight zone.

It's true that high-performance athletes, who train for several hours every day and use the latest exercise equipment to track their heart rate, lactic acid threshold, and metabolic rate, can benefit from Zone 2 training—particularly when it's used in combination with intense interval training. But for the purposes of longevity, you get a lot more bang for your buck with other types of cardio. So save yourself from the numbers and statistics, the monitors and blood tests—obsessing over the zone of your training intensity is not going to make you any healthier. At the end of the day, just find a type of cardio that you like to do, do it for a minimum of 75 minutes per week, and don't worry about what zone you are in!

The second type of exercise—**strength training**, or weight lifting—should be done to increase and maintain muscle mass. Muscle mass only slightly declines—about 3% per year— from age 30 until about age 60, when it begins to decline more rapidly. It really starts to plummet after about age 60 and in severe cases can lead to a loss of about 50% of total muscle mass by the 8th and 9th decades of life. While it is inevitable to lose some muscle mass as you age, "short-term muscle inactivity severely reduces muscle mass and strength even in young individuals." Thus, strength-training exercises help reduce the rate of decline, keeping people stronger longer into old age. You don't have to pump iron or get a gym membership for strength training. You can add muscle to your arms and shoulders by doing push-ups and pull-ups or pulling on resistance bands. Ever notice how those swimmers have V-shaped bodies? That tells you they are getting plenty of strength training in their arms, shoulders, and backs while swimming laps. You can add muscle to your lower body by performing squats, climbing stairs, walking uphill, cycling, skating, and even dancing. Also, shoveling in the garden strengthens muscles.

The last type of essential exercise is **balance and flexibility training**. Anyone with young children knows that we lose flexibility and range of motion as we age. Our joints just aren't as pliable as those of children. Kids can do the splits or seemingly fold themselves in half. No wonder champion gymnasts are so young—they depend on that childhood flexibility. People also lose balance as they age. The key to balance is a strong core—those abdominal and back muscles.

Want to retain both balance and flexibility? The best answer is yoga. Those down dogs, lunges, lizards, warriors, triangles, pyramids, planks, pigeons, and tree poses are the simplest way to develop—and keep—both flexibility and balance. For most of my adult life, I didn't practice yoga. Like a lot of people my age I thought, it seemed, I don't know, not like real exercise. But then my running partner told me about his yoga class, which was filled with older people who were more flexible and had better balance than he did. So, I decided to attend an introductory class, expecting it to be a breeze. Boy, was I wrong. It was hard work. The next week I went back and felt so much better after. Eventually, it became a routine. These days, the opportunities to try out yoga are legion; studios are everywhere.

But you don't have to go to a studio or take an organized class to stretch and balance. There are plenty of stretching instructions and guided yoga videos on the Internet. Or you can even just stretch at home on your own. Just settle on a set of exercises—touching your toes, doing squats and lunges, bringing your foot to your behind to stretch your quads— make up your own routine. Just be sure you incorporate all the main muscle groups—quads, hamstrings, ankles, hips and glutes, shoulders, neck, wrists, and the rest. Even just 5 to 10 minutes a day can keep you limber with a routine that is easy to stick to.

Some activities tick off two or even three exercise types at once. For example, swimming is both muscle strengthening and aerobic: Doing laps can help you build muscles as well as heart and lung capacity. Vinyasa yoga, a dynamic flowing style of yoga, may test your balance and flexibility as well as your aerobic capacity. But the big winner that hits all three types of exercise—aerobic, muscle strengthening, and balance and flexibility—is cross-country skiing. The people who, by certain measures, are in the best shape in the world are mostly Norwegian cross-country skiers. These dual- or triple-action activities may be a good investment of time to keep you strong and healthy into old age.

But not all sports are equally beneficial. Golf is immensely popular but hardly exercise. It is more of a social game, like bocce ball or croquet. A comprehensive review of studies on golf showed, first, that using a golf cart negates most benefi-cial effects associated with the physical activity of golf. A cart makes golf a virtually sedentary activity, only a bit better than watching it on TV from an exercise standpoint. About two-thirds of American golfers routinely use golf carts and thus get no exercise value from 3 to 4 hours on the course. They might get social value or a dose of sunshine, but no aerobic or strength-training value.

Even when you walk and haul your own golf bag, golf does not provide any vigorous level of physical activity. While some argue that "golf *can* provide moderate intensity physical activ-ity," that sneaky word "can" means it is far from a ringing endorsement. Indeed, carrying your own bag 18 holes is low-intensity physical activity, especially when spread across the 3 to 4 hours it takes to finish 18 holes. In other words, as the reviewers put it, "golfers may find it difficult to play enough during a week in order to reach recommendations [for 150 minutes of moderate activity] and may wish to supplement golf with another [exercise]." So, a weekly golf game is not really a form of moderate exercise. Golf with a cart has the same energy expenditure as croquet . . . and mopping the floor. Aiming for wellness and longevity? Try riding a bike before hitting the course.

Many people get plenty of exercise from playing football, ice hockey, rugby, and other heavy-contact sports. They defi-nitely can enhance aerobic activity and build strength and muscle mass. And of course, engaging in these sports may provide satisfaction and social engagement. But the health dangers they pose outweigh the benefits. Specifically, these sports all involve significant risk of serious head injuries. That is why I don't recommend playing them for exercise. The risk of smashing your head is too high, and your head is the most valuable thing you have!

There are some animals that have evolved over millennia to take repeated head smashing. Think woodpeckers. But humans are not woodpeckers. Even minor head trauma in humans can cause concussions, and the cumulative effect of repetitive impacts to your head leads to brain damage. As I noted in Chapter 3, the technical term for this type of brain damage is chronic traumatic encephalopathy, or CTE. A growing body of evidence from sports players shows that repeated head injury kills brain cells, leading to emotional and mood disorders, behavior problems, and dementia. It can also lead to drug abuse, overdoses, and suicide. Not consistent with wellness or longevity.

A chilling article about this recently appeared in a leading medical journal. The researchers examined and dissected the brains of young athletes who had engaged in amateur football, hockey, soccer, rugby, and wrestling and had suddenly died. Among the 152 young athletes, with an average age of roughly 23, a staggering 41% were found to have CTE. Even more concerning, the most common cause of death among these athletes was suicide, followed by unintentional overdose. Another recent study of 77 professional or amateur ice hockey players who died showed that nearly all—96%—had CTE. Worse, there was what researchers call a dose response—the more years played, the worse the CTE. About 20% of players who skated for less than 13 years had CTE, which increased to over 50% for those who played 13 to 23 years, and 96% for those who played over 23 years.

It's true that football, rugby, and other contact sports can provide useful skills besides exercise: teamwork, discipline, perseverance. But as valuable as these skills are, they can all be obtained without such a high risk of smashing your brain. Good alternatives include volleyball, baseball, and swimming.

So, if you want to be well, forgo the head-smashing sports. And if you have children and want *them* to be well, consider not letting them engage in such sports, which are not going to promote their health or long life. Of course, every family has the right to follow its own discretion, and any parent must make hard choices when faced with a child's decision to engage in high-risk behaviors. But think of it this way. Convincing a child *not* to start smoking, for example, could mean they get an extra 10 years—and healthy ones, too. Similarly, convincing a child *not* to play football is likely to significantly reduce their chances of serious brain injury.

While exercise is essential to good health, there is a limit to its benefits. The CDC recommends at least 150 minutes per week (about 20 minutes per day) of moderate exercise or 75 minutes per week (about 10 minutes per day) of vigorous exercise. But are these recommendations just a minimum? Do the health benefits of exercise continue to increase the more you exercise?

Yes and no. A long-term, 30-year follow-up study of over 100,000 doctors and nurses found that health improvements increased with more exercise. Compared with people who did not exercise at all, those who engaged in 150 to 300 minutes of moderate activity per week or 75 to 150 minutes of vigorous activity per week had a 19–25% lower risk of death from all causes, including both cardiovascular and noncardiovascular (for example, cancer) disease. Notably, exercising more than the recommended amount further reduced deaths, but there was what the economists call diminishing returns. Compared with people who got 75 to 150 minutes of vigorous activity per week, people who did 150–300 minutes showed a meager 4% additional decrease in premature deaths. Similarly, people doing 300 to 600 minutes (5 to 10 hours) per week of moderate exercise—2 to 4 times the minimum—showed a 3–13% additional decrease in premature deaths.

Beyond 300 minutes per week of vigorous exercise or 600 minutes per week of moderate exercise, there were no additional improvements. Importantly, there didn't seem to be any harm either—more exercise did not lead to more deaths. But at 10 hours per week of exercise, you are certainly sacrificing time spent in other valuable activities, like talking to your friends or giving back to your community.

The upshot: You get the most health benefits by going from horizontal to some moderate physical activity. Then you get progressively more health benefits—and a decline in deaths—by exercising up to about 10 minutes per day vigorously or 20 minutes per day moderately—that is, 75 minutes per week vigorously or 150 minutes per week moderately. But beyond that threshold, there are only small impacts on mortality. Exercising 2 or 3 hours a day will not improve your longevity more than 45 minutes a day.

There are two potential downsides of exercise: injuries and sudden death. Every person who regularly exercises inevitably sustains an injury. Some types of physical activity are more injury prone than others. For instance, running increases the risk of injuries more than walking or hiking. Biking can also be dangerous—I'm still recovering from a recent bike spill, which seems to occur every other year or so. This one was my worst accident yet, leaving me with two fractured ribs, a nondisplaced pelvic fracture, and torn ligaments in my shoulder. I narrowly avoided a direct head smash, thanks to my helmet. But it was sufficiently bad that, uncharacteristically, I took a couple of days off of work and actually saw a physician who ordered some X-rays! I, too, am a "good" doctor who avoids engagement with the medical system as much as possible. But this time I couldn't.

The risks of exercise are real. But here are five precautions that can reduce the risk and severity of injuries:

- First, wear protective equipment. This is an easy one. My helmet certainly prevented a serious concussion or worse, and there is plenty of evidence that "helmets decrease the potential for severe traumatic brain injury following a collision by reducing the acceleration of the head upon impact." A meta-analysis of 55 studies conducted over the last 35 years showed that "the use of bicycle helmets was found to reduce head injury by 48%, serious head injury by 60% and traumatic brain injury by 53%, and face injury by 23%." Indeed, head injuries and deaths decline when helmets are made mandatory. So be sure to wear a helmet when bicycling, skating, or skiing.
- Second, focus on your flexibility and balance—not only because it is independently valuable, but because it may also help prevent injury. Stretching by itself will not make you immune to injury; in fact, "there is moderate to strong evidence that routine application of static stretching does not reduce overall injury rates." However, there is growing but not definitive evidence that static stretching does reduce muscle and tendon injuries. More high-quality research is needed on the impact of dynamic stretches before exercise.

What to do? A few experts summed up the situation this way: "The relationship between stretching and injury risk remains controversial. The answer to 'can I stretch?' is yes—it probably will not increase injury risk. But the answer to 'do I have to stretch?' is 'possibly no'—as the likelihood of decreasing the injury risk is contentious."Arguably the best advice is that an enduring practice of yoga or other flexibility and balance training does not *cause* injuries and may also help *prevent* exercise-induced injuries. This effect is in addition to the benefits of improving flexibility and balance.

- Third, warm up. Before any exercise session, warm up for 10 to 15 minutes to increase your heart rate, prepare your metabolism for work, and heat up your muscles. Start with some dynamic movement, focusing on the muscles you will be using. Begin your activity slowly and mindfully, allowing your body to adjust before increasing the intensity. A recent review of 15 studies showed a 36% reduction in sports injuries among children and adolescents while using a structured warm-up routine. Similarly, warming up is good for the heart, especially for people who are at risk for heart disease. There is even a name for it: "warm-up angina." Some people experience chest pain when initiating exercise, as the heart's oxygen demand exceeds supply. But after the brief initial effort, the heart undergoes physiological changes that increase its blood flow and prepare it for exercise. The post-warm-up effort is then less likely to cause chest pain or changes in an electrocardiogram reflecting insufficient blood supply to the heart. The initial warm-up not only dilates vessels and recruits collateral vessels to improve the blood flow to the heart, but also increases the heart's resistance to low oxygen levels and improves the efficiency of each heartbeat. This phenomenon has been noted for at least two centuries. So warm up before intense exercise to reduce injuries and heart problems.
- Fourth, cross-train. Space out and vary your workouts so you don't get repetitive-motion injuries by overdoing it with the same muscle group. Shin splints, tennis elbow, swimmer's shoulder, and runner's knee can often be avoided if you allow your body to recover between efforts. Even leaving

just a day or two between intense workouts, or alternating running with weight training and swimming, allows time for those minor muscle tears and bone strains to heal while you are exerting other muscle groups.

- Fifth, don't rush the recovery. Exercise fanatics inevitably want to get back to exercising after an injury. They feel deficient or unfulfilled if they don't run or swim or bicycle while injured. But not letting the body fully heal risks creating chronic problems. Take, for example, ankle sprains, the most common foot and ankle injury in sports. Research shows that taking the time to properly rehabilitate the ankle with functional exercises, through at-home exercises or supervised physical therapy, decreases risk of reinjury. The importance of rest only increases for more serious injuries, like anterior cruciate ligament (ACL) tears. One study showed that individuals who return to strenuous activity before the recommended 9-month mark had a 7 times increased likelihood of reinjuring their ACL compared with those who waited.

I have to admit this is still a work in progress for me. My very first question to the doctor examining me after my bike accident was "When can I start riding again?" A few years ago, after another bike accident, I insisted on cycling to the emergency room despite bleeding from a puncture wound. I understand the difficulty of waiting for recovery—but I also recognize its importance. This time, to allow my body to heal, I waited 4 full months after the accident and made sure to start with a gentle 15-mile ride.

My best advice for recovery is the adoption of cross-training. For example, if you sprained your ankle while running, but still feel the need to exercise, then switch to an exercise that does not use your legs, such as upper-body weight lifting or swimming without kicking.

In addition to these tips to reduce the frequency and severity of injury, remember: *Don't be a schmuck!* Avoid self-destructive risks whenever possible. If you're going on a run, hike, bike ride, skiing expedition, or open water swim, tell a friend or family member where you are going and when you'll be back. Check the weather and dress appropriately—I have been caught too many times underdressed for biking in a strong wind or hiking above the tree line in a sudden downpour. Finally, be visible by using reflective clothes and lights.

Aside from injuries, exercise can also increase your risk of sudden death during and just after exertion. One of my college roommates, a member of our college's cross-country team and a lifelong runner, dropped dead while running at age 37. Sudden death is almost always a cardiac event. For younger athletes—those under 35—the main cause of sudden cardiac death is a genetic or congenital defect in the heart's structure, like abnormally thick walls of the left ventricle. For older athletes, the biggest risk is a heart attack (blockage in the coronary arteries) or an arrhythmia (electrical malfunction). Though the thought of these events is frightening, the actual risk is incredibly low. A 19-year study of high school athletes in Minnesota showed that the risk was about 1 in 400,000 to 1 in 900,000. That's basically 4 athletes out of 1.6 million students who participated in at least one sport.

Obviously, this exercise-induced risk is much higher for people who exercise infrequently and much lower for habitual exercisers who have improved their aerobic function. Furthermore, the risk is strongly associated with extreme exercise, like marathons. However, from the data collected between 2010 and 2023, the risk of having a heart attack during a marathon or half marathon is exceedingly low: about 1 in 200,000. Dying of a heart attack during a marathon is even lower: 1 in

500,000. That is comparable to being struck by lightning in a 2-year period. Very, very rare.

The most important takeaway about exercise and sudden death is that the associated health benefits way, way, way outweigh the small risk. But there is a peak to the health benefits of exercise. So it is important not to overdo this good activity.

While you should be careful not to overdo exercise, it is also important to keep it up. As with many of the activities of wellness, exercise is a paradigmatic case of "use it or lose it." Everybody will have to skip a workout once in a while or even take a break from exercise or heal from an injury. But don't let that break last too long. Otherwise, you will become deconditioned, quickly losing all the physiological advantages of exercising.

Anyone who has taken a break from exercising for a long vacation or major work or family obligation can confirm that these improvements dissipate quickly. The cardiac advantages begin to diminish in a few days and are really gone within 4 weeks. Just 2 months without exercise will lead to reduced muscle mass and muscle strength. And there are other changes when you stop exercising: Higher blood pressure and worse management of blood glucose start within days, and accumulated benefits can be gone in just weeks of no exercise. All of these negative impacts of exercise cessation manifest more rapidly and severely as you age.

Give yourself permission to skip a workout or two, but don't make it a habit. Make aerobic exercises, strength training, and yoga part of your daily or weekly routine. That is the right exercise cocktail for life. As you age, maintaining your exercise routine becomes even more crucial.

How anyone makes exercise a routine depends on their personality. Just as I don't follow any particular diet but simply eat well, I also exercise for wellness and longevity without obsessing about numbers or times. I find success in keeping up pleasurable exercises, eventually turning them into a habit. But my wife is different. She is motivated by her workout numbers, probably because she went to MIT, where it seems everyone focuses on numbers. She looks at how many steps she takes every day, her speed and distance biking, and her $\dot{V}O_2$ max. If you, like my wife, feel better when you can assess your performance, there are two main physiological indicators of wellness and longevity. One relates to aerobic exercise and the other to strength.

The first indicator is $\dot{V}O_2$ max, which is a measure of a person's maximum ability to consume oxygen assessed at peak performance. The absolute highest $\dot{V}O_2$ max numbers ever recorded are between 90 and 97.5. They tend to be predominantly among professional cyclists and cross-country skiers, although for some reason, there is disproportionate representation of Norwegians among athletes with the best $\dot{V}O_2$ max. Results from a 2020 study on over 11,500 treadmill assessments across the United States, Canada, and Norway found that men in their 20s have a median $\dot{V}O_2$ max of about 50 and women in their 20s have a median of about 41. Higher numbers are strongly associated with physical capacity and longevity. Conversely, lower $\dot{V}O_2$ max is associated with a much higher risk of dying. As one article put it: "VO_2max is one of the most predictive biometrics for cardiovascular health and overall mortality."

Unfortunately, $\dot{V}O_2$ max declines precipitously with age— about 9% per decade. A $\dot{V}O_2$ max of 50 in a 25-year-old man typically drops down to about 31 in his 70s. And a $\dot{V}O_2$ max of 41 in a 25-year-old woman typically drops down to 25 in her 70s. Importantly, by engaging in aerobic exercise—running, cycling, rowing, hiking, and the like—especially as you age—

you can raise your $\dot{V}O_2$ max to that of a young person and physically do more. So keep up that exercise and you will have found the $\dot{V}O_2$ max fountain of youth.

Note that directly and accurately measuring $\dot{V}O_2$ max is complicated and requires a sports lab, where you run on a treadmill or ride a stationary bike hooked up to EKG monitor and a mask that precisely measures your inhaled and exhaled oxygen and carbon dioxide. I have never had a lab measure my $\dot{V}O_2$ max, but rely on the fair assessments on phone apps and fitness trackers. They estimate your maximum heart rate and use a formula such as 15.3 $\times$ (maximum HR/resting HR) to calculate your $\dot{V}O_2$ max. Since we rarely go all out and hit our maximum heart rate during routine exercise sessions, these $\dot{V}O_2$ max estimates are on the low end.

The second essential biological predictor of mortality and longevity is grip strength. As a major study in 17 countries with nearly 150,000 people concluded: "Grip strength was inversely associated with all-cause mortality, cardiovascular mortality, non-cardiovascular mortality, myocardial infarctions, and stroke." That is, the greater your grip strength, the lower your mortality risk. This probably has little to do with the strength in our hands and arms and more to do with overall frailty and lack of full-body conditioning. Amazingly, our hands have become significantly weaker since 1985, probably because we do less farming and manufacturing, shoveling and digging. Instead, we do more sitting at desks and on couches, typing on our computers, and therefore are overall not as well conditioned.

Nevertheless, you can improve your grip strength by doing all sorts of strength training and by squeezing tennis or rubber balls, doing dead hangs from bars in the gym, or doing exercises with free weights like bicep curls. Try to incorporate grip strength exercises as part of your muscle-building program.

———

The most important lesson is that you just need to do *some* regular exercise, something you enjoy that can become part of your routine. From the perspective of wellness and longevity, exercise need not become your life. There is a plateau to the benefits. Work yourself up to 75 minutes of vigorous exercise a week (10 to 15 minutes a day) and eventually up to the sweet spot of 150 minutes per week. And ensure that you do the three kinds of exercise—aerobic, strength, and balance and flexibility training. All are important to your wellness and longevity, especially as you age. And don't smash your head in the process, please—brain damage would certainly spoil all your hard work for wellness.

6

Sleep Like a Baby

Getting the Rest You Need

In high school, I had a debate partner who used to complain about how much time he was wasting on sleep. He calculated that sleeping 8 hours a day meant that a third of his life was wasted doing nothing. "Wasted" was his exact word.

This type A attitude has pervaded society, including the field of medicine. For at least the last century, health systems have scheduled doctors to work overnight and forgo sleep in order to care for their sick patients. As a resident physician in the 1950s, my father spent almost three years of his life on call every other night. This meant that across each two-day period, he worked about 36 hours straight, followed by 12 hours for sleeping and "the rest of life." Even in the 1980s, when I was a medical resident, we still had a few every-other-night on-call shifts—typically when we were in the intensive care units with the sickest patients. By that time, though, schedules had largely moved to the "luxurious" every third night on call. This meant we worked for 36 hours, were off for 12 hours, back for 10 to 12 hours on the third day, and left to fit "the rest of life"—including sleep—into the remaining 12 to 14 hours. Sleep deprivation was just part of life.

This might have been excusable when I was in medical school 40 years ago. Back then, we knew next to nothing about sleep. At my medical school, I recall only a few details from our very few lectures on sleep: something about REM sleep and dreaming, the presence of slow-wave sleep, and the fact that big herbivores like elephants need to stay awake longer than smaller ones to have enough time to eat. (This is true of herbivores but not carnivores.) But the purpose of spending one-third of a lifetime on sleep was still largely a mystery. Hence, lots of smart people I knew, like my debate partner, were actively trying to sleep less in order to get more done.

It turns out that the "sleep is a waste of time" attitude is flat-out wrong. The simplest refutation of this opinion is the fact that humans do, in fact, sleep for one-third of their lives. Nothing that leaves an animal unconscious, defenseless, and exposed to myriad dangers would have been conserved over the millions of years of mammalian history and tens of thousands of years of human evolution if it was not absolutely essential.

Indeed, over the last few decades we have learned that sleep is a fundamental aspect of wellness, health, and longevity. Lack of sleep is associated with numerous negative health effects, including heart disease, obesity, type 2 diabetes, high blood pressure, and even cancer. In a detailed study on the impact of bad sleep patterns on health, researchers at the Beth Israel Hospital in Boston followed 172,000 adult Americans for an average of 4.3 years and linked them to the National Death Index. People who experienced five characteristics of bad sleep—short sleep time, trouble falling asleep, trouble staying asleep, waking up in the night, and taking medications to fall asleep—were more than twice as likely to suffer from significant obesity, type 2 diabetes, and heart disease and 1.5 times as likely to get cancer. And a British study involving data from over 400,000 individuals investigated the link between sleep and cardiovascular outcomes. Self-reported short sleep (at most 5 hours) was associated with a 25% higher risk of overall mortality and a 27% higher risk of cardiovascular mortality.

Why does sleep matter for chronic disease? One possible explanation is that sleep deprivation seems to cause immune system dysfunction. For instance, it lowers antibody production in response to the flu vaccine, reducing its effectiveness. Bad sleep patterns are also linked to other underlying physiological problems, such as metabolic dysfunction, inflammation, increased fight-or-flight responses, and other changes that altogether increase the risk of developing chronic diseases.

Not only does short and bad sleep lead to poorer health, but it actually causes premature death. In an older meta-analysis of 16 different studies involving nearly 1.4 million people, researchers found that shorter sleep was associated with greater risk of death. And those Beth Israel researchers showed that even after controlling for the other things we know can cause death, like smoking, having good-quality sleep of sufficient duration was strongly associated with fewer deaths. Indeed, for the 172,000 people in their study, they calculated that having good sleep was associated with an extra 4.7 years of life for men and 2.4 years for women. That is *huge*.

It also turns out that short and disrupted sleep is associated with some things we all dread: bad decision-making, cognitive impairment and dementia. Acute sleep deprivation has an immediate detrimental impact on cognitive ability, while chronic sleep deprivation can raise your long-term chances of developing dementia. In the short term, impairments from acute sleep deprivation are like being intoxicated. Studies have found that staying awake for 17 hours causes a similar impact on your functional abilities as having a blood alcohol level of 0.05%—what is technically called being "buzzed." You may experience minor impairment of reasoning and memory and exaggerated emotions. Pulling an all-nighter—that is, staying awake for at least 24 straight hours—is like having a blood alcohol level of 0.1%, equivalent to being legally drunk, with impairments of balance, speech, vision, and, most importantly, slow reaction times, reduced self-control, and poor judgment. As the National Institute for Occupational Safety and Health puts it: "Sleep deprivation impairs your information processing and learning. Both short-term recall and working memory decline." That means you cannot remember simple things like an address or that you have to call someone. This also leads to bad risk assessments and an increase in risk-taking behaviors.

Just being sleep deprived for 24 hours can be deadly in some circumstances. Sleep deprivation for doctors and nurses is linked to patient dissatisfaction, medical errors, and patient deaths. One study of over 11,000 physicians found that "moderate, high, and very high sleep-related impairment were associated with 53%, 96%, and 97% greater odds of self-reported clinically significant medical error." And lots of disasters may be partially due to sleep deprivation. Think about the Space Shuttle *Challenger*, which exploded 73 seconds into its flight, partly because those who authorized liftoff made the judgment call without sleeping the previous night. Too many airplane, bus, and truck accidents are also linked to sleep deprivation.

Beyond the immediate cognitive impairment and risk, there are also long-term impacts of consistently poor sleep. The most worrisome finding is that chronic sleep deprivation increases the risk of dementia. A study by Charles A. Czeisler, the Baldino Professor of Sleep Medicine at Harvard and one of my old medical school professors, followed over 2,800 older adults in good health. Participants who reported consistently short sleep times—less than 5 hours—and poor-quality sleep—such as taking over 15 minutes to fall asleep—were at significantly higher risk for developing dementia. Indeed, seniors who slept less than 5 hours a night were twice as likely to get dementia.

Similarly, researchers in Finland followed over 2,300 Finnish twins over age 65 for an average of 22 years. They recorded their sleep characteristics and use of sleep medications. Seniors who slept under 7 hours per night scored lower on cognitive tests. And those with poor sleep quality also had lower cognitive function. The researchers concluded that "[poor] sleep related characteristics may emerge as a new risk factor for cognitive impairment." Similarly, a recent study of more than 2,800 teenagers showed that insufficient sleep adversely affected the decision-making parts of the brain and behavior control.

So not only is my old debate partner destined for a sicker and shorter life than he might otherwise have had, but he's also more likely to experience cognitive limitations and dementia as he ages.

Why is sleep so important—especially to cognitive function? Our best understanding today is that sleep facilitates many essential functions, most of which have to do with keeping the brain clean, healthy, and in top shape. First, sleep allows the brain to process the day's input. An important part of this sleep-induced processing is brain cell "reorganization"—that is, making new connections with other brain cells that reflect the day's activity. Another part of that processing helps us form memories. Sleep allows short-term memories lodged in the hippocampus to consolidate into long-term memories in the prefrontal cortex. In addition, sleep allows the body to clean up brain waste. As your brain carries out its essential functions throughout the day, it naturally produces toxic by-products—garbage. Just like in a city, garbage accumulation in the brain is noxious and harmful. When asleep, the brain can clean out garbage that would inhibit proper functioning.

In the brain and beyond, sleep serves an important restorative purpose. Namely, sleep facilitates the repair and growth of many cells in the body, including brain and stem cells. This is one reason parents swear their babies "grew overnight." The multiplication of those stem cells means kids really do grow as they sleep!

What makes us feel tired and ultimately fall asleep? Many people think melatonin is the secret. Not true. The real sleep substance is the neurotransmitter adenosine. Throughout the day, adenosine accumulates in the brain, causing people to become less alert and shift into sleep mode. While asleep, adenosine levels gradually fall, allowing you to wake up refreshed and alert.

We can interfere with this adenosine cycle in a number of ways. Caffeine keeps us alert by blocking adenosine receptors, preventing fatigue and sleep. Napping will also reduce adenosine levels—that is how naps make us more alert. Though caffeine and naps can help increase alertness and focus during the day, the resulting adenosine blockage or reduction can diminish the drive for nighttime sleep. Understanding the role of adenosine in inducing sleep can help us figure out how to improve our sleep: avoiding caffeine intake at least 6 to 7 hours before bedtime and minimizing naps, especially from the mid-afternoon on.

But how much sleep do we need? And when should we be sleeping? Getting 7 to 8 hours of sleep is a good rule of thumb. However, it is an average. The optimal amount of sleep across the board is a bell-shaped curve, with the majority of people needing 7 to 8 hours. Some people are naturally short-sleepers and can function normally on 6 or even fewer hours. Some people skew in the other direction, needing more than 10 hours of sleep to function normally. If you feel tempted to say you're a short- or long-sleeper, it's possible but statistically unlikely; the number of true short- and long-sleepers is very small. It's better to assume you're like most of us who need 7 to 8 hours.

To determine how much sleep you actually need, give yourself a weeklong test. Go to bed when you feel sleepy, not just tired. That will reduce the time it takes to fall asleep. And don't set an alarm, just wake up naturally. After a week, you will be able to determine how much sleep you need to be alert and function normally without the need to drink coffee all day or take naps.

Once you know how much you should sleep every night, prioritize it. Don't be a schmuck like my old debate partner and think that sleep is optional. The most important step is to make consistent sleep part of your routine.

Finally, it is a myth that you need less sleep as you age. As we get older, we may well sleep less because of a decrease in deep, slow-wave sleep and a tendency to wake up more often. But that is different from *needing* less sleep. To get the right amount as you age, you may need to supplement nighttime sleep with a nap.

Just as people naturally need different amounts of sleep, people also may need to sleep at slightly different times. I once invited Frances M. Kamm, the Henry Rutgers University Professor of Philosophy at Rutgers, to be a yearlong visiting scholar in my NIH bioethics department. She accepted, but with one condition: no requirement to show up any day before 2 p.m. and the ability to work in the office until 2 or 3 in the morning. I readily agreed, but with one condition of my own. Every year, we spend one day selecting the following year's pre- and post-doctoral fellows, and we wanted her to attend because we val-

ued her judgment. By long tradition, the meeting would start at
8:30 a.m. and last through most of the day. After a long silence,
she said, "Alright, I guess I'll just stay up all night that day."

A chronotype describes the natural pattern of one's sleep/
wake cycles, whether you are a night owl or an early bird.
Clearly, Kamm is a night owl. Over the years, I have found that
most journalists I know are night owls, while most surgeons
are early birds.

What are you? Do you get out of bed early or do you have
a tendency to stay up late and then sleep in? My two brothers are early birds. They tend to be awake and exercising at
5:30 a.m. (Actually, Ari is awake and working out at 4:30 a.m.
I have been the recipient of too many calls when I am barely
conscious on the East Coast while he is pumping iron in Los
Angeles.) If you do the weeklong test without an alarm, you
will also figure out if you are an early bird or a night owl.

If you are an early bird, you are sleepy in the afternoon and
need to be in bed before about 9 p.m. Be sure you don't schedule too many important meetings or try to make big decisions
in the late afternoon or evening—that is the time you will have
less energy and mental focus. Also don't attend lots of late-
night parties. Get home early enough to go to bed and have a
good night's sleep.

If you are a night owl, then make sure your mornings are
clear—or as E. E. Cummings supposedly said when he was a
college student, "No classes before 10 a.m." Being a night owl
might allow you to work better when those early birds are
snoozing in bed and the house or office is quiet. But, like Fran-
cis Kamm, you might need a more flexible work environment
that allows you to come in and stay later. And in the spirit of
improving your wellness holistically, you might also have to
be more deliberate about exercise, since studies show that
night owls tend to work out less than early birds.

Importantly, chronotype does not determine how much sleep you need—the overall amount of sleep is different from the timing of when you go to sleep and wake up. Be sure you respect both characteristics of your sleep pattern.

As a wellness behavior, sleep is unique. It is different from eating well or exercising or even having strong social relationships. You can will yourself to drink less soda or to hop on the bike or even talk to the cashier at the grocery store. But you cannot get into bed and force yourself to get high-quality sleep. The biggest problem with urging people to sleep more is that our willpower cannot make sleep happen.

Nevertheless, there are seven things you can do that increase the chances you will get restful sleep. These things can help, but cannot guarantee, a good night's sleep. They are often called "sleep hygiene"—a term I hate because it sounds like sanitation. Instead, let's call it the road to better sleep:

- First, make your bedroom conducive to sleep. Keep it dark and cover up all those red, green, blue, and white lights on various electronic items—or just take them out of your bedroom. Exposure to light at night can disturb your circadian rhythm. Also keep your bedroom cool. We sleep better at lower temperatures, between 62° and 65° Fahrenheit.
- Second, figure out your caffeine tolerance. Caffeine works by blocking adenosine receptors in the brain, preventing adenosine's sleep-inducing function. Some people are not kept awake by caffeine. But for most of us, caffeine encourages wakefulness. While each person's metabolism is different, the half-life of caffeine (how long it takes for the initial concentration of caffeine in the bloodstream to drop in half) is 3 to 7 hours, though the range can be as large as 1.5 to 9 hours. Thus, have your last coffee or tea—or, if you must, caffeinated

soda—at least 7 hours before your usual bedtime. I tend to have my last cup of caffeinated tea before noon and then switch to herbal teas or other noncaffeinated drinks like apple cider.

- Third, avoid alcohol close to bedtime. Most people think alcohol helps them fall asleep. And while it does slow brain activity, depresses the nervous system, and induces relaxation, it is not an insomnia cure. Because alcohol is a short-acting drug (it takes 1 hour to metabolize 1 drink), it can make falling asleep easier but actually make it harder to stay asleep, thereby diminishing the quality and total amount of sleep. Alcohol shortens REM sleep, which is important for memory consolidation. This may be one reason drinkers often don't remember what you told them the night before. But it also has a tendency to disrupt and fragment sleep, making it more likely you will wake up during the night, resulting in less overall sleep. The less alcohol rule for eating well is one you should also adopt for improved sleep.
- Fourth, don't doomscroll or otherwise engage your electronics (computer, tablet, or phone) for an hour before bed. Screens emit blue light that interferes with your circadian rhythm and melatonin release. And one thing I have learned the hard way: If you leave your phone on or don't put it in sleep mode, the random buzzing text message from a family member in another time zone can interrupt your beauty rest.

My routine is to put my phone in another room on sleep mode. I brush my teeth and otherwise get ready for bed. In bed, I read a book—one printed on paper. (It is shown we retain more of the content when we read books on paper.) And when I find myself finishing a paragraph with heavy eyelids, I know it is time to put the book aside, turn off the light, and go to sleep.

- Fifth, make sure to exercise regularly and eat fruits, vegetables, and whole grains. Exercise not only directly improves wellness and longevity, but can help indirectly by improving sleep quality. It improves both REM and slow-wave sleep. A study found that eating more fruits, vegetables, and whole grains during the day improved sleep quality by 16% at night. Meditation, relaxation techniques, and mindfulness exercises before bed can also improve sleep. These are not sleep aids that can be simply switched on and off. They take practice and consistent use until they become a habit. But if you are patient and work at them for a few months, they can give you years of benefit.

- Sixth, don't nap after 2 p.m. Napping after lunch for 10 to 30 minutes can make you mentally sharper in the afternoon. But napping after 2 p.m. disrupts the accumulation of adenosine necessary for sleep and can delay the onset of sleep at night.

- And seventh, avoid staring at the clock during the night. Cover the clock, turn the clock around, leave your phone in the kitchen. Any kind of mental activity can keep you up or increase the time it takes to fall asleep. Who cares what time it is when you wake up in the middle of the night before your alarm clock goes off?

For those with more persistent insomnia, these seven tips might not be enough to ensure restful sleep. But be wary of looking to the pharmacy for help. Existing sleep medications suck. They might be able to give us some shut-eye, but generally fail at giving us the deep, restorative sleep that is so important for health, wellness, and longevity. You would be perfectly logical in thinking that a great sleeping pill might be one loaded with adenosine. Unfortunately, adenosine administered as a medication cannot cross the blood-brain barrier to effectively increase brain levels. Hence, there is no adenosine sleeping pill.

Some people think melatonin is the magical sleep substance. With the onset of nighttime darkness, melatonin is naturally secreted from the pineal gland into the bloodstream. Melatonin decreases signals from the circadian clock that keep us alert and synchronize our sleep/wake cycle. This can be useful for people with jet lag or on night shifts to help shift the sleep schedule.

But melatonin is not the true sleep substance. Hence, it is controversial whether melatonin helps healthy adults who have difficulty falling and staying asleep. The American Academy of Sleep Medicine does not recommend taking melatonin for either sleep onset or maintenance, but acknowledges that conclusive evidence is weak. For some people a melatonin pill at night—no more than 5 milligrams for adults—may help induce sleep. Whether it truly works or is an effective placebo, we don't know for sure. And be careful in selecting your supplement. Lots of melatonin pills on the market don't contain the quantity of melatonin they list. But at 5 milligrams, there are relatively few side effects, so experimenting to see if it helps you may be reasonable.

There are many other sleeping pills. The evidence for their effectiveness in either promoting sleep onset or maintaining sleep is, as the American Academy of Sleep Medicine put it, weak. And according to the Cleveland Clinic, "Studies show that sleeping pills aren't that helpful in promoting a good night's rest." You might fall asleep a few minutes faster or experience longer sleep duration—but it is generally not good-quality sleep. And all of these pills have side effects, including feeling mentally foggy the next day—precisely the feeling you were trying to avoid with restful sleep.

Instead of taking sleeping pills, it is better to identify and fix the root cause of your sleeplessness. So, if you are having trouble falling asleep or staying asleep, or if you can't keep your eyes open during the day, let your primary care doctor know before the issue goes on for too long. Problems with sleep can be due to medical or psychiatric problems, other medications you are taking, or a specific sleep disorder such as sleep apnea.

The most effective intervention for sleep problems is cognitive behavioral therapy for insomnia (CBT-I). It typically involves working with a psychologist or therapist to focus on feelings and thoughts leading to insomnia and implementing the seven techniques to better sleep, such as relaxation and meditation, no caffeine near bedtime, exercise, and fruits and vegetables. Data suggest that the majority of patients who pursue this treatment approach improve. And the American College of Physicians recommends CBT-I as a first-line treatment for insomnia. There are two main reasons people don't often use this treatment. First, there is a shortage of psychologists and therapists trained in CBT-I. Second, we live in a quick-fix society where people hesitate to put in the time to learn how to fall asleep again. These problems, though, don't change the fact CBT-I is the safest and most effective way to treat insomnia, way safer and more effective than "sleeping pills."

Millions of people are using sleep trackers to improve their sleep. This is a mistake. Unlike sleep lab studies, these consumer trackers, like Oura Rings, Fitbit, WHOOP, or Apple Watches, don't measure sleep directly, but rather infer it from body motion, heart rate, temperature, and blood oxygen levels. While they have gotten more accurate, within 90–95% of lab values in distinguishing sleep versus wake states, they tend to underestimate the number of times a person wakes and overestimate total sleep time by registering inactive wake time as sleep. These misclassifications cause the individual to overlook their fragmented sleep pattern. In general, these monitors have significant difficulty distinguishing the various stages of sleep. They tend to underestimate deep sleep and accurately categorize sleep stages only 50–85% of the time. Sometimes they even fail to record an entire actual night of sleep. In one study, for instance, the Apple watch failed to record a night's sleep about 17% of the time. Overall, at the time of writing this book, the Oura Ring appears to be the most accurate. While these sleep trackers may provide some information, they cannot be used to identify or diagnose real sleep problems.

But the real issue with sleep trackers, along with the surplus of dubiously accurate information they provide, is that they can just make you more anxious. Becoming obsessed by the numbers cannot induce better sleep and may do just the opposite. Indeed, this worry about the sleep numbers even has a name: "orthosomnia." As one physician put it, "The most accurate measure of good sleep is how you feel upon waking," not what the numbers say. By fixating on the sleep numbers generated by wearables, people can easily become anxious and stressed. This does not help with either falling asleep or getting a good night's rest. Remember that you cannot will yourself to have a good night's sleep. All you can do is "make the bed"—follow the specific recommendations to prioritize getting the right amount of sleep and follow a regular routine that increases the chances of falling asleep. It is much, much better to forget what the sleep tracker "tells" you and listen to your body's natural cues.

Getting a good night's rest can be a challenge, but increasing your odds of sleeping well is relatively simple. Prioritize getting sleep within your busy life. Figure out how much sleep you need. Try to figure out your chronotype to determine when you are the most productive. And follow the proven methods that are known to increase good sleep.

Afterword

Be a Mensch

Being healthy and living long does not require extreme religious devotion or heroic sacrifice. In fact, a wellness *obsession* tends to cause anxiety and frustration—which are definitively anti-wellness. The goal is to integrate healthy behaviors into the fabric of your everyday life so they become automatic and easy, not a chore, burden, or all-consuming fixation.

Making changes to your routines will improve your health and wellness, but remember that you don't need to be perfect. It's not necessary to score 100% in each area to decrease your risk of developing disability and dementia or to have a long, healthy, fulfilling life. Having a soda (or, in my case, a piece of my mother's cheesecake), missing a few days or weeks of exercise, temporarily skimping on sleep to complete an important project—none of these lapses is going to make you unhealthy or measurably reduce the length of your life. More importantly, occasionally not following one of the behaviors can make you feel better. I once was with one of the world's leading longevity experts, who told me that an optimal diet could add 5 years to one's life, but then said, "I'm going to enjoy this bacon, which I guarantee is not part of an optimal diet." Wellness is not any single choice or action. It is not maximizing any single behavior, but the cumulation of years and decades of the right lifestyle. As we all know, no life is perfect. We all slip up occasionally. That's okay. The important aspect is that these deviations are exceptions and not your norm. They should be occasional and last a relatively short time. Be a mensch. Forgive yourself for these infrequent digressions and return to your routine.

There are three other important wellness messages worth making explicit. First, the pervasive notion that wellness is all about the physical—eating, exercising, and sleeping—is wrong. In popular culture, the most important wellness and longevity behaviors—the social and mental—are forgotten or deemphasized in favor of the physical. But remember this: Cultivating social relations and staying mentally engaged are even more important than eating well or exercising.

The distressing thing is that these essential wellness behaviors are threatened by the trappings of our modern era. All the time we spend on smartphones and social media is time not spent engaging with people face-to-face. Being with other people—eating with them, exercising with them, volunteering with them, and just talking with them about anything at all, even briefly—is the most important thing you can do for wellness as well as happiness.

Supercentenarians are those very rare people who live to 110 years or longer. To get to 110, a person has to be essentially well, avoiding disability and cognitive impairment. How do they do it? Undeniably, a large part of it is genetics. We can't change that . . . at least not yet. But interviews with supercentenarians reveal common practices that we can all adopt. Some of these older adults pump iron in the gym. Others swear by a good diet . . . or scotch. But the factor they most commonly cite is family, friends, and social relations. As one Australian supercentenarian says: "Family is for me, everything." Another advises: "Always remember to be kind to yourself and others too. . . . I always try and be helpful to others in everything that I do, I try to put a smile on someone's face." Christian Mortensen, an American who lived to 115 years and 252 days, shared his wellness secrets: "Friends, a good cigar, drinking lots of good water, no alcohol, staying positive and lots of singing will keep you alive for a long time." Similarly, a study of people who lived to 100 in Hong Kong found that "all participants, regardless of their living arrangements, reported to have positive relationships with others, especially with younger family members and neighbors. All have maintained frequent contact with their family members. For the three participants who lived alone, they were visited by their children or grandchildren almost every day." Interviews with people who lived to 100 are replete with similar remarks about the importance of family, friends, and engaging with others.

Robust social connections are important for the *quality* of one's life in addition to its *length*. A study of undergraduates found that the happier ones were those who "were highly social, and had stronger romantic and other social relationships." These students reportedly "did not exercise significantly more, participate in religious activities significantly more, or experience more objectively defined good events," yet were still happier. These findings strongly support the necessity of social relationships for happiness. If there is one wellness behavior to focus on it is family, friends, and social relations—not just to extend your life but to enrich it.

It turns out that there is something called the "well-being paradox" in Latin American countries. Many Latin American countries have high happiness and emotional well-being, yet they have high social, political, and economic challenges. Latin Americans tend to be happier than their per-person national income would predict. The most likely explanation is that they are incredibly social and have the world's highest frequency of shared meals with family and friends, on average more than 8 per week.

Interestingly, prioritizing social relations doesn't occur in a vacuum. When pursued as a facet of a fulfilling life, forming and maintaining social relationships inevitably involves other wellness behaviors. Having friends over for a home-cooked meal, walking with your neighbor, riding in a cycling studio with others, taking a language class, or joining a book club are ways to maintain and enrich your friendships, meet new friends who share your passion, and elevate your acquaintances to genuine friends. They are also ways to eat well, exercise regularly, and keep mentally sharp.

This brings us to the second important message: There is a "wholeness" to wellness behaviors. Wellness is really a lifestyle made up of overlapping patterns of behavior, all of which reinforce each other and together create forward momentum toward a long, fulfilling life. Helpful ways to get high-quality sleep are to exercise during the day, eat a healthy diet of fruits and vegetables, forgo caffeine or alcohol before bed, and avoid looking at your computer or screens an hour before bed. Scheduling early-morning workouts reduces the likelihood you will stay out late drinking. Exercising with a friend helps incentivize the repetitions necessary to make exercise a habit. Having social support is important for avoiding harmful triggers and breaking those high-risk habits like smoking. Engaging in wellness behaviors such as exercising, sleeping well, and talking to friends are effective ways to manage stress.

Each wellness behavior supports the others and makes living healthy more automatic. When you get all six wellness behaviors reflexively integrated into your life, you will be at your healthiest and happiest.

My third and most important message is this: Wellness and living long are only a means to a good life. They are not, themselves, the essence of a good life, as so many influencers and wellness gurus make them out to be. An unfulfilling life, no matter how long and healthy, is not the ideal. It will cause more suffering than satisfaction. A long life is worthwhile only if it is filled with meaningful relationships and activities. These wellness practices should enhance the best parts of your life and allow you to more fully enjoy the activities and people you love for many years to come.

I hope that you will enjoy the process of incorporating wellness into your life. You should *enjoy* being in nature when you run or bike or hike. You should *enjoy* a delicious healthy meal with your family or close friends. You should *enjoy* expanding your mind through conversations with friends, interesting books, and new experiences. But despite enjoying these activities, they should not become the focus or the purpose of your life. Spending your time fixated on how to efficiently maximize $\dot{V}O_2$ or increase your grip strength, how to get the most hours of quality sleep, or counting exactly how many ounces of meat you are eating is a mistake. Be a mensch. Keep sight of the *reasons* you want to live longer. Don't just try to accumulate years of life without appreciating their value. In the end, you will regret it.

One of the best people for advice on leading a fulfilling and long life—and not regretting having wasted precious time—is Benjamin Franklin. After all, he lived to 84 years of age in an era when the average life expectancy was about 36. More importantly, he lived a life filled with achievements, friends,

scientific discoveries, and social contributions. He was mentally sharp and engaged right up to the last days of his life.
Franklin would tell you to do three things: keep challenging
yourself and constantly improve, devote yourself to friends
and acquaintances, and commit yourself to making the world
a better place. Or as he might summarize it, "be useful."

As a young man, Franklin created a moral diary with 13 virtues and assessed how he improved on them each week. As an
older man, he recognized his prejudices and flaws and worked
on overcoming them. Franklin corresponded with over 1,000
people, back when that involved writing long, formal letters,
not firing off a quick email. He routinely dined with others
at clubs, coffee shops, and pubs. To be useful, Franklin constantly created social groups and unions. He organized a club
of craftsmen who sought education and self-improvement, as
well as a group of subscribers to create a lending library. He
created a fire brigade, the Pennsylvania Hospital, the University of Pennsylvania, and several other organizations to
improve life in Philadelphia, the United States, and the world.
He conducted electrical experiments with like-minded amateur scientists. And he created the American Philosophical Society for people to gather and exchange new ideas and
advance human knowledge. He did for others, he enjoyed his
pursuits, and he was useful. We all have different talents and
different ways of being useful, but the key is to use those talents to do good for others. All the data show that activities in
the service of others make us happier and more fulfilled.

Franklin was not against making money, but he was
against greed. For him, money was only good if it served the
purpose of improving his community and the wider world—
not to pile ever higher for himself. Franklin was not opposed
to enjoying life, but he was against making the maximization
of pleasure the central focus. I imagine that Franklin would

have felt similarly about longevity. Accumulating years of life is not an independently meaningful objective. It is how you use those years—the positive change you can make with the time you have.

Most importantly, Franklin was not a perfectionist. He understood that we all make mistakes and have flaws. But with them lie opportunities for growth. It is essential to acknowledge our limitations and grow. We can continually improve and overcome our mistakes, prejudices, and errors. Franklin would have advised: Figure out what you want to devote yourself to, who you want to befriend, and ultimately, what you want to be remembered for when your life ends. And he did say: "Be at war with your vices, at peace with your neighbors, and let every new year find you a better man"—or woman.

Don't make living forever the purpose of your existence. Happiness and health come as by-products of a meaningful life. They naturally fall into place as part of the wholeness of being well.

Start thinking like Franklin and figure out what you can do to be useful. Health, wellness, and longevity will follow.

Acknowledgments

This book has many sources. Several years ago at a conference, Ariana Huffington asked me why medical education did not include more information on wellness. Her question prompted me to delineate six wellness behaviors and make the argument that there was little incentive to push for more medical and nursing education on wellness because none of the big health care institutions—insurers, hospitals, drug companies, or clinicians—would make a lot of money from wellness. Her question was astute and important, but I felt I was too busy, and didn't write anything . . . yet.

At the end of 2023, I read one of the seemingly endless books being published by the wellness-industrial complex. It infuriated me. It emphasized exercise, with smaller sections on diet and sleep—totally leaving out social relationships and mental engagement. Furthermore, many of its recommendations were unproven—even unprovable—and were so detailed and untested that they probably would not add minutes, much less weeks or months, to a person's life, but would take up a lot of time. Ultimately, the real thing that incensed me was the increasing tendency of all wellness commentators and gurus to make wellness into a kind of religion, make it the end goal rather than just a means that fades into the background while people pursue the valuable activities that make life meaningful. Yes, like riding a bike in the beautiful countryside or cooking and sharing a delicious meal with friends, wellness should be enjoyable and enhance life, not be obsessive drudgery. Obsessively thinking about it, the way these books and newsletters induce you to do, struck me, as my father would say, as "being a schmuck."

There is nothing like being pissed off to get someone to pick up the pen. In three weeks, I scribbled the first draft of this book. It might have never seen the light of day but for two people: Kara Swisher and Adam Grant. Kara was being interviewed at Penn by Adam, and then we went out for dinner. When the conversation turned to what I was working on, I mentioned the wellness manuscript I had written but put aside. They both encouraged me—well, did way more than encourage me—to finish and publish it, saying that Americans needed an antidote to the gym rats and wellness mindset. They even went so far as to introduce me to their publishers, agents, PR teams, and others who could help—all the time insisting that I not put the book on the back burner.

Then, in 2024, I refined it, and in early 2025 did a final revision. As people heard I was writing this along the way, I was prompted by many friends and acquaintances to include additional material, alter recommendations, and make other improvements.

That is a long way of saying that I owe a debt to many people that this book did not end up as a manuscript collecting dust at the bottom of some desk drawer.

Importantly, there were many experts who generously read

different chapters and saved me from errors while adding critical points that I had ignored or overlooked or simply did not know about. What is remarkable is that many of them did not know me or owe me anything before I cold-called or emailed them asking for their advice and criticism. Nevertheless, they all freely gave of their time and knowledge to ensure that my information on wellness was accurate.

I greatly appreciate the huge amount of uncompensated, careful editorial work of so many: Marion Nestle, Corby Kummer, Mark Hyman, and Steve Nissen read the chapter on eating well and offered many criticisms. We don't agree on everything—like potatoes—but they offered numerous insights and corrections. The former surgeon general, Vivek Murthy, offered important corrections for the chapter on social relationships, including the point that made me further research the negative impacts of just having cell phones face down on a table. This led me to revise the chapter but also ban cell phones from my classrooms to improve focus and actual enjoyment of the interactions—and it worked for students. Similarly, Robin Dunbar provided useful comments on friendships. And Gillian Sandstrom answered my out-of-the-blue email with helpful guidance related to research on and the value of weak interactions. Also, thanks to my good friend Katie Hafner for allowing me to quote an illustrative passage from her book *The Boys.*

Angela Duckworth, Katy Milkman, and Michael Inzlicht gave me useful advice on willpower, emphasizing the difference between it being a limited resource and being easily fatigued. Gil Welch gave me great advice on the cancer screening section, encouraging me to acknowledge the burdens of uncertainty, worry, and having to hassle with the health care system from overdiagnosis. Chuck Czeisler and Charles Bae helped enormously with the sleep chapter. The exercise chapter was greatly improved by Jonathan Mitchell, particularly telling me about the original study of London bus drivers and conductors from the 1950s. Susann Rohwedder, an expert on the impact of retirement on cognitive abilities, helped me with the chapter about mental sharpness. And Michael Meyer gave me some obscure but very helpful information about Benjamin Franklin.

Of course, none of these people who "answered the call" from no one they knew bear any responsibility for any errors that may appear in this book. All the mistakes are mine alone, especially since I did not always take their advice.

Thanks to Johan Dellgren, Merjan Ozisik, Sam Lopez-Rico, Patricia Hong, and Danielle Brown, my research assistants, who did a mountain of work and lost lots of sleep and often chided me about many of my wellness suggestions. They tirelessly and very effectively found studies I didn't know about, criticized my prose—or dull sentences—corrected my grammar, suggested additions, put the citations in a proper order, and everything else necessary for a book. They made this book so, so much better.

Also, thanks to my administrative assistants—Angela Golub, Betsy Straw, and Hannah Malloy—who scheduled me and rescheduled me when I double and triple booked myself and, most importantly, found me sufficient writing time in a crazily packed schedule to make sure I could complete the book.

For many years, I have received sage advice from my agent Suzanne Gluck. She has worked with me on those important academic books that few people would read. But she pushed me to make this wellness book more personal and helpful and, most importantly, accessible and enjoyable so the widest possible audience would actually learn from it. Dara Kaye was a new agent on my case, helping me with the book proposal and book. But her sense of humor saved the day when she changed the title. I always wanted it to be *Don't Be a Schmuck*, but she realized that the real positive messages were contained in *Eat Your Ice Cream*.

Matt Weiland is my new editor at W. W. Norton. He read and scribbled over several chapters, helping me recognize how to make the book even more accessible by elaborating important research without giving in to my tendency to weigh the prose down with too much data. He also encouraged me to be more personal and also to be frank about the importance of not being too hard on yourself, not trying for what might be thought of as "wellness perfection." He made sure that I emphasized that one key to wellness was getting it right most of the time but allowing yourself a few non-wellness indulgences. Those are not going to shorten your life by minutes, much less days or weeks, and they add variety and make life fun. I love to bake, and the cakes and cookies and crostatas add richness to my life even if they are not on any wellness diet.

I want to express my great appreciation to my copyeditor, Janet Greenblatt. Copyeditors rarely get acknowledged, but Janet made numerous corrections that made the book flow better and encouraged me to consider myriad changes to clarify my arguments and examples. This book is much, much better because of her scrupulous work.

Finally, there is my family. My wife Teasel is endlessly supportive of all my hairbrained ideas and even claims she enjoys participating in them. I cannot thank her enough for not only putting up with me, but doing yoga with me every morning even when we are apart by doing the exercises via shared video, riding our bikes together through the countryside, and nursing me when I seem to inevitably injure myself. Her help on this book was enormous: critiquing some of my suggestions, helping me rephrase ideas, editing my sentences and chapters, and not letting me give up. She wanted this book to be perfect, and however close it comes is in large measure attributable to her indefatigable help with every aspect of it.

And, thanks to my daughters, who are among my harshest critics. (They have a tough competition from Teasel and my brothers.) Everyone needs some people who will tell them the unvarnished, unfiltered truth, forcefully. They read chapters, giving suggestions, criticisms, and ideas. I always appreciate their astute comments and ability to cut to the core.

I also need to thank one of my sons-in-law, Benjamin Armstrong, who carefully read the book and offered important suggestions, especially around behavior change and willpower . . . many of which I took.

Finally, there are my brothers—they are endlessly supportive while being incredibly critical—a most helpful combination. They, too, lived with my father—and learned how not to be schmucks, but work for justice, speak their minds, and enjoy meeting people.

Rahm is the model of steadiness on wellness—the model of regular exercise, sleeping and eating well, and mental engagement by reading books and articles. Over many, many years, Ari constantly calls me with questions about various tests and treatments that might improve wellness, health, and longevity. He is great at exploring the complete wellness universe, talking to experts on all continents, and being the guinea pig for anything that he assures himself won't kill him. He has introduced me to a multitude of crazy ideas, sent me numerous wellness concoctions and other things to try—from rat parasites to inversion tables to supplements. Honestly, I don't necessarily consume them all . . . but he never gives up. What I love about him is that while he pursues wellness, it never crowds out the other rich aspects of his life.

In many ways, working on this book has been a huge part of wellness. It forced me to engage with my family and a wide group of friends and find new experts to learn from. My fervent hope is that everyone can figure out how to adopt wellness behaviors and focus on leading rich, multifaceted lives with the few years we have on this amazing planet.

Notes

Introduction

2 **"Drinking is not really beneficial to your health":** Pierre Ducimetiere et al., "Coronary Heart Disease in Middle-Aged Frenchmen: Comparisons Between Paris Prospective Study, Seven Countries Study, and Pooling Project," *The Lancet* 315, no. 8182 (June 1980): 1346–50; M. H. Criqui and B. L. Ringel, "Does Diet or Alcohol Explain the French Paradox?," *The Lancet* 344, no. 8939 (December 1994): 1719–23; Richard D. Semba et al., "Resveratrol Levels and All-Cause Mortality in Older Community-Dwelling Adults," *JAMA Internal Medicine* 174, no. 7 (July 2014): 1077–84; Sohaib Haseeb, Bryce Alexander, and Adrian Baranchuk, "Wine and Cardiovascular Health: A Comprehensive Review," *Circulation* 136, no. 15 (October 2017).

3 **As Thoreau eloquently summarized:** Henry David Thoreau, *Walden: Or, Life in the Woods* (Ticknor and Fields, 1854).

5 **While some studies:** Deborah J. W. Lee, Ajla Hodzic Kuerec, and Andrea B. Maier, "Targeting Ageing with Rapamycin and Its Derivatives in Humans: A Systematic Review," *The Lancet Healthy Longevity* 5, no. 2 (February 2024): E152–62.

5 **This extrapolation of laboratory findings:** Karen Brown et al., "Resveratrol for the Management of Human Health: How Far Have We Come? A Systematic Review of Resveratrol Clinical Trials to Highlight Gaps and Opportunities," *International Journal of Molecular Sciences* 25, no. 2 (January 2024): 747.

6 **"Our only goal":** Peter Attia, *Outlive: The Science and Art of Living Longer* (Harmony Books, 2023).

6 **Life expectancy on the eve:** "Life Expectancy (from Birth) in the United States, from 1860 to 2020," Statista, last modified August 9, 2024.

6 **Today, even with the problems:** Sherry L. Murphy et al., "Mortality in the United States, 2023," NCHS Data Brief no. 521 (December 2024).

6 **Wellness was launched:** Daniela Blei, "The False Promises of Wellness Culture," *JSTOR Daily*, January 4, 2017.

7 **Dr. Means's book:** Nicholas Florko, "Casey Means, Trump's Surgeon-General Nominee, Has a Lot in Common with RFK Jr.," *The Atlantic*, May 2025.

8 **Even the teachings of Hippocrates:** Carl J. Lavie, James H. O'Keefe, and Robert E. Sallis, "Exercise and the Heart—The Harm of Too Little and Too Much," *Current Sports Medicine Reports* 14, no. 2 (March/April 2015): 104–9.

8 **At about the same time, Aristotle devoted:** Attributed to Aristotle, *Aristotle, XIX, Nicomachean Ethics*, 2nd ed., trans. H. Rackham (Harvard University Press, 1934).

8 **Risk management, friendship:** Office of the Surgeon General (OSG), *Our Epidemic of Loneliness and Isolation: The U.S. Surgeon General's Advisory on the Healing Effects of Social Connection and Community* (US Department of Health and Human Services, 2023).

10 **"Happiness is not a goal":** Attributed to Eleanor Roosevelt, *You Learn by Living: Eleven Keys for a More Fulfilling Life*, reprint ed. (Harper Perennial, 2016).

10 **It can lead to long-term inflammation:** Agnese Mariotti, "The Effects of Chronic Stress on Health: New Insights into the Molecular Mechanisms of Brain–Body Communication," *Future Science OA* 1, no. 3 (November 2015).

10 **They just live rich, healthy lives:** Dan Buettner, *The Blue Zones: Lessons for Living Longer from the People Who've Lived the Longest*, illustrated edition (National Geographic, 2010); Dana G. Smith, "Do People in 'Blue Zones' Actually Live Longer?," *New York Times*, October 24, 2024, sec. Well.

11 **longer and healthier lives:** There is controversy regarding the accuracy of reported ages and the reliability of data sources. Critics' claims have not been substantiated in peer-reviewed articles, while the ages have been cross-checked from multiple sources and substantiated in many cases by one of the world's best and most respected demographers and longevity experts, Michel Poulain.

11 **Nor am I offering:** Eric Topol, "The Business of Promoting Longevity and Healthspan," Substack newsletter, *Ground Truths* (blog), March 22, 2025.

13 **Milkman and her colleagues:** Hengchen Dai et al., "The Impact of Time at Work and Time Off from Work on Rule Compliance: The Case of Hand Hygiene in Healthcare," The Wharton School Research Paper, no. 56 (September 2014), available at SSRN.

14 **"prior exertion of of self-control":** Bastien Blain, Guillaume Hollard, and Mathias Pessiglione, "Neural Mechanisms Underlying the Impact of Day-long Cognitive Work on Economic Decisions," *Proceedings of the National Academy of Sciences* 113, no. 25 (June 2016): 6967–72.

14 **"I judg'd it would be":** Benjamin Franklin, *Benjamin Franklin's Autobiography: A Norton Critical Edition*, ed. Joyce E. Chaplin (W.W. Norton, 2012).

16 **Some lore:** Benjamin Gardner, Phillippa Lally, and Jane Wardle, "Making Health Habitual: The Psychology of 'Habit-Formation' and General Practice," *British Journal of General Practice* 62, no. 605 (December 2012): 664–66.

16 **Others claim 66 days:** Phillippa Lally et al., "How Are Habits Formed: Modelling Habit Formation in the Real World," *European Journal of Social Psychology* 40, no. 6 (October 2010): 998–1009.

16 **James Clear, of *Atomic Habits*:** James Clear, "How Long Does It Actu-

ally Take to Form a New Habit? (Backed by Science)," *James Clear* (blog), March 6, 2014.

17 **Micro or tiny changes:** Jeanette Brown, "10 Tiny Habits That Spark Massive Life Changes," *Global English Editing*, March 7, 2025.

17 **For example, a recent study:** Anne-Julie Tessier et al., "Consumption of Olive Oil and Diet Quality and Risk of Dementia-Related Death." *JAMA Network Open* 7, no. 5 (May 2024): e2410021.

19 **"We defeat death":** "Rosh Hashanah Family Edition," Jonathan Sacks: The Rabbi Sacks Legacy, accessed April 2025.

Chapter 1: Don't Be a Schmuck

23 **As scootering becomes:** Adrian N. Fernandez et al., "Injuries with Electric Vs Conventional Scooters and Bicycles," *JAMA Network Open* 7, no. 7 (July 2024): e242413.

24 **I *would* tell you:** "Tobacco Use Among Children and Teens," American Lung Association, last modified November 12, 2024.

24 **Indeed, the habit is so nasty:** "Smoking Cessation: Fast Facts," CDC: Smoking and Tobacco Use, September 13, 2024.

24 **Because, on average, a smoker:** Richard Doll et al., "Mortality in Relation to Smoking: 50 Years' Observations on Male British Doctors," *BMJ* 328 (June 2004): 1519.

24 **and a heavy smoker:** "Heavy Smokers Cut Their Lifespan by 13 Years on Average," Statistics Netherlands, September 15, 2017.

24 **Each cigarette a smoker lights up:** Sarah E. Jackson, Martin J. Jarvis, and Robert West, "The Price of a Cigarette: 20 Minutes of Life?," *Addiction* 120, no. 5 (May 2025): 810–12.

24 **Quitting by age 44:** Prabhat Jha et al., "21st-Century Hazards of Smoking and Benefits of Cessation in the United States," *New England Journal of Medicine* 368, no. 4 (January 2013): 341–50.

24 **In 2024, researchers in South Korea:** Jun Hwan Cho et al., "Smoking Cessation and Incident Cardiovascular Disease," *JAMA Network Open* 7, no. 11 (November 2024): e2442639.

25 **He was a four-pack-a-day:** Michael Merschel,"The Presidential Heart Attack That Changed America," American Heart Association News, February 15, 2024.

25 **One day in 1949:** Stephen E. Ambrose, *Eisenhower Volume I: Soldier, General of the Army, President-Elect, 1890–1952* (Simon & Schuster, 1985).

25 **"The President then told me":** "Eisenhower Gives Tip On Quitting Cigarettes," *New York Times*, January 31, 1964, sec. Archives.

25 **Despite decades of smoking:** "Table V.A3 Period Life Expectancies, Calendar Years 1940–2001," Social Security Online, Office of the Chief Actuary, last modified April 9, 2002.

25 **In fact, it has long been thought:** Michael Chaiton et al., "Estimating the Number of Quit Attempts It Takes to Quit Smoking Successfully in a Longitudinal Cohort of Smokers," *BMJ Open* 6, no. 6 (June 2016): e011045.

26 **More recently, Canadian researchers:** Chaiton et al, "Estimating the Number of Quit Attempts."

26 **One proven strategy involves:** Anna E. Mazzucco, "Quitting Smoking: Women and Men May Do It Differently," National Center for Health Research, January 12, 2015.

26 **But maybe the most important thing:** Mazzucco, "Quitting Smoking."

27 **A recent analysis of 90 research trials:** Nicola Lindson et al., "Electronic Cigarettes for Smoking Cessation," *Cochrane Database of Systematic Reviews*, 1, no. 1 (January 2025).

27 **Hence, the British government supports:** Andy McEwen et al., "Vaping: A Guide for Health and Social Care Professionals," National Centre for Smoking Cessation and Training, last modified November 2023.

27 **However, the FDA:** "Vaping and Quitting," CDC: Smoking and Tobacco Use, August 27, 2024.

27 **And after reviewing the data:** US Preventive Services Task Force, "Interventions for Tobacco Smoking Cessation in Adults, Including Pregnant Persons," *JAMA* 325, no. 3 (January 2021): 265–79.

27 **Surprisingly, that was the same percentage:** John P. Pierce et al., "Role of E-Cigarettes and Pharmacotherapy During Attempts to Quit Cigarette Smoking: The PATH Study 2013–16," *PLOS ONE* 15, no. 9 (September 2020): e0237938.

27 **And the study was repeated:** Yadira Galindo, "Studies: E-Cigarettes Don't Help Smokers Quit and They May Become Addicted to Vaping," UC San Diego Health, September 2, 2020; Ruifeng Chen et al., "Use of Electronic Cigarettes to Aid Long-Term Smoking Cessation in the United States: Prospective Evidence from the PATH Cohort Study," *American Journal of Epidemiology* 189, no. 12 (December 2020): 1529–37.

27 **Even worse, a subsequent study:** Natalie E. Quach et al., "Daily or Nondaily Vaping and Smoking Cessation Among Smokers," *JAMA Network Open* 8, no. 3 (March 2025): e250089.

28 **Vaping hit a boom:** Rob Stein, "Surgeon General Warns Youth Vaping Is Now an 'Epidemic,'" NPR, December 18, 2018, sec. Public Health.

28 **The next year, youth vaping peaked:** Teresa W. Wang et al., "Tobacco Product Use and Associated Factors Among Middle and High School Students—United States, 2019," *MMWR Surveillance Summaries* 68, no. 12 (December 2019): 1–22, CDC.

28 **Luckily, the federal and state crackdown:** "E-Cigarette Use Among Youth," CDC: Smoking and Tobacco Use, October 17, 2024.

28 **"Between 2019 and 2023":** Anjel Vahratian et al., "Electronic Cigarette Use Among Adults in the United States, 2019–2023," NCHS Data Brief no. 524 (January 2025), Centers for Disease Control and Prevention.

28 **A 2017 review:** Samir Soneji et al., "Association Between Initial Use of E-Cigarettes and Subsequent Cigarette Smoking Among Adolescents and Young Adults: A Systematic Review and Meta-Analysis," *JAMA Pediatrics* 171, no. 8 (August 2017): 788–97.

29 **Michael Blaha, director:** Michael Joseph Blaha, "Will Vaping Lead Teens to Smoking Cigarettes?," Johns Hopkins Medicine, Wellness and Prevention, August 29, 2024; John Erhabor, Zhiqi Yao, Erfan Tasdighi, Emelia J. Benjamin, Aruni Bhatnagar, Michael J. Blaha, et al., "E-cigarette Use and Incident Cardiometabolic Conditions in the All of Us Research Program," *Nicotine & Tobacco Research*, March 15, 2025; "New Analysis Underscores Health Risks of E-Cigarettes," Johns Hopkins Medicine, April 15, 2025

29 **Emphasizing this point:** "Changes to Vaping Rules in Australia," Alcohol and Drug Foundation, October 21, 2024.

29 **A recent study showed that college students:** American Neurological

Association, "Vaping Bad for Brain Health, First-of-Its Kind Study Shows," Newswise, September 15, 2024.

29 **And like cigarettes:** Francesco Versace, Ph.D, "Vaping and Your Brain: What to Know," University of Texas MD Anderson Cancer Center, April 19, 2024.

30 **The highest use:** Rachel Nania, "1 in 5 Older Adults Uses Cannabis," AARP, September 12, 2024.

31 **Since legalization:** Kusum Adhikari, Alexander Maas, and Andres Trujillo-Barrera, "Revisiting the Effect of Recreational Marijuana on Traffic Fatalities," *International Journal of Drug Policy* 115 (May 2023): 104000.

31 **For moms there is increased risk:** Kelly C. Young-Wolff, Sara R. Adams, Stacey E. Alexeeff, et al., "Prenatal Cannabis Use and Maternal Pregnancy Outcomes," *JAMA Internal Medicine* 184, no. 9 (July 22, 2024): 1083–93.

31 **brain development problems:** Sophia Badowski and Graeme Smith, "Cannabis Use During Pregnancy and Postpartum," *Canadian Family Physician* 66, no. 2 (February 2020): 98–103.

32 **"Long-term cannabis users showed":** Madeline H. Meier, Avshalom Caspi, Annchen R. Knodt, Wayne Hall, Antony Ambler, HonaLee Harrington, et al., "Long-Term Cannabis Use and Cognitive Reserves and Hippocampal Volume in Midlife," *American Journal of Psychiatry* 179, no. 5 (May 2022).

32 **Heavy drinking:** "Alcohol Use and Your Health," CDC: Alcohol Use, January 14, 2025.

32 **"the 10th most relevant":** "Alcohol Use," Institute for Health Metrics and Evaluation, accessed March 9, 2025.

32 **In 2020, alcohol was:** Dana Bryazka et al., "Population-Level Risks of Alcohol Consumption by Amount, Geography, Age, Sex, and Year: A Systematic Analysis for the Global Burden of Disease Study 2020," *The Lancet* 400, no. 10347 (July 2022): 185–235.

33 **They reported, however:** "Alcohol Use," IHME.

33 **For instance, a British study:** Rosario Ortolá et al., "Alcohol Consumption Patterns and Mortality Among Older Adults with Health-Related or Socioeconomic Risk Factors," *JAMA Network Open* 7, no. 8 (August 2024): e2424495.

33 **The positive impact:** Kenechukwu Mezue et al., "Reduced Stress-Related Neural Network Activity Mediates the Effect of Alcohol on Cardiovascular Risk," *Journal of the American College of Cardiology* 81, no. 24 (June 2023): 2315–25.

33 **"There are no studies that would":** Benjamin O. Anderson et al., "Health and Cancer Risks Associated with Low Levels of Alcohol Consumption," *The Lancet Public Health* 8, no. 1 (January 2023): e6–7.

33 **After all, alcohol is causally linked:** Béatrice Secretan et al., "A Review of Human Carcinogens—Part E: Tobacco, Areca Nut, Alcohol, Coal Smoke, and Salted Fish," *The Lancet Oncology* 10, no. 11 (November 2009): 1033–34; Harriet Rumgay et al., "Global Burden of Cancer in 2020 Attributable to Alcohol Consumption: A Population-Based Study," *The Lancet Oncology* 22, no. 8 (August 2021): 1071–80.

33 **Ultimately, both WHO:** "No Level of Alcohol Consumption Is Safe for Our Health," World Health Organization Europe, January 4, 2023; "UK Chief Medical Officers' Low Risk Drinking Guidelines," Department of Health, GOV.UK, August 2016.

34 **Every month, 1.2% of adults:** "Impaired Driving Facts," CDC: Impaired Driving, October 18, 2024.

34 **Further, the CDC's data:** "Impaired Driving Facts," CDC.

34 **At the federal blood alcohol limit:** "Drunk Driving," National Highway Traffic Safety Administration, accessed March 13, 2025.

34 **Indeed, even for blood alcohol levels:** "Reaching Zero: Actions to Eliminate Alcohol-Impaired Driving," National Transportation Safety Board Safety Report, May 14, 2013.

35 **Every 39 minutes:** "Drunk Driving," NHTSA.

35 **If you drink:** Christopher R. Conner et al., "Association of Rideshare Use with Alcohol-Associated Motor Vehicle Crash Trauma," *JAMA Surgery* 156, no. 8 (August 2021): 731–38.

35 **fatalities, and DUI convictions:** Michael L. Anderson and Lucas W. Davis, "Uber and Alcohol-Related Traffic Fatalities," Working Paper 29071 (July 2021), National Bureau of Economic Research; Charles Hughes, "Study: Ride-Sharing Reduces Traffic Deaths and DUI Arrests," *The Federalist*, June 16, 2016.

35 **Texting while driving:** "Driver Distraction in Commercial Vehicle Operations," Federal Motor Carrier Safety Administration, US Department of Transportation, September 2009.

35 **In 2010 the National Safety Council:** "National Safety Council Estimates That At Least 1.6 Million Crashes Are Caused Each Year by Drivers Using Cell Phones and Texting," PR Newswire, January 10, 2010.

35 **In 2019, nearly 425,000 people:** "Distracted Driving," CDC: Distracted Driving, May 16, 2024.

35 **All driving deaths dropped:** "Historical Fatality Trends: Car Crash Deaths and Rates," National Safety Council Injury Facts, accessed March 13, 2025.

36 **Furthermore, decreased exposure to sunlight:** G. W. Lambert et al., "Effect of Sunlight and Season on Serotonin Turnover in the Brain," *The Lancet* 360, no. 9348 (December 2002): 1840–42.

36 **We all need at least:** "The Health Benefits of Sunshine (and How Much You Need Per Day)," Cleveland Clinic, February 20, 2025.

36 **The sun streaming through our eyes:** "The Health Benefits of Sunshine," Cleveland Clinic.

36 **Sunlight on our skin:** "The Health Benefits of Sunshine," Cleveland Clinic.

36 **Too much sunlight:** "Cancer Causes and Prevention, Risk Factors: Sunlight," National Cancer Institute, National Institutes of Health, April 26, 2023.

36 **Randomized and population studies:** Reza Ghiasvand et al., "Sunscreen Use and Subsequent Melanoma Risk: A Population-Based Cohort Study," *Journal of Clinical Oncology* 34, no. 33 (November 2016): 3976–83.

36 **Misinformation on TikTok:** Sandee LaMotte, "Social Media's Message About the Sun and Sunscreen: 'It's Frightening,'" CNNHealth, June 21, 2024.

36 **"52% of Gen Z adults":** "American Academy of Dermatology Survey Shows Gen Z Adults at Risk for Skin Cancer Due to Increasing Rates of Tanning and Burning," American Academy of Dermatology, May 14, 2024.

36 **"getting a tan was more important":** "American Academy of Dermatology Survey," AAD.

36 **Another survey by a cancer institute:** "Survey Finds Young Adults More Likely to Believe Myths About Sun Protection and Skin Cancer Prevention," Orlando Health, May 1, 2024.

37 **Some of the concerns:** Anahad O'Connor, "The Claim: A Sunscreen Chemical Can Have Toxic Side Effects," *New York Times*, June 13, 2011, sec. Health; NCTR Technical Report E02186.01, National Toxicology Program, US Department of Health and Human Services, June 23, 2016.

37 **And you would have to use sunscreen:** Steven Q. Wang, Mark E. Burnett, and Henry W. Lim, "Safety of Oxybenzone: Putting Numbers into Perspective," *Archives of Dermatology* 147, no. 7 (July 2011): 865–66.

37 **You can easily avoid:** Elisabeth Anderson and Joe Zagorski, "Trending—Mineral Sunscreen," Michigan State University Center for Research on Ingredient Safety, May 6, 2024.

37 **And dying of melanoma:** Maurie Markman, "Metastatic Melanoma," City of Hope, June 20, 2022.

37 **A 2007 review found:** The International Agency for Research on Cancer Working Group on artificial ultraviolet (UV) light and skin cancer, "The Association of Use of Sunbeds with Cutaneous Malignant Melanoma and Other Skin Cancers: A Systematic Review," *International Journal of Cancer* 120, no. 5 (March 2007): 1116–22.

37 **"using tanning beds before age 20":** Seokyung An et al., "Indoor Tanning and the Risk of Overall and Early-Onset Melanoma and Non-Melanoma Skin Cancer: Systematic Review and Meta-Analysis," *Cancers* 13, no. 23 (November 2021): 5940.

37 **And did I mention that UVA:** "10 Surprising Facts About Indoor Tanning," American Academy of Dermatology Association, last modified April 26, 2023; Verena Reimann et al., "Sunbed Use Induces the Photoaging-Associated Mitochondrial Common Deletion," *Journal of Investigative Dermatology* 128, no. 5 (May 2008): 1294–97.

37 **Moreover, tanning salons:** "10 Surprising Facts about Indoor Tanning," AAD.

38 **Vaccines have allowed us:** "Smallpox," Countdown to Zero, American Museum of Natural History, accessed March 14, 2025.

38 **Polio is also:** "About Global Polio Eradication," CDC: Global Polio Vaccination, September 10, 2024.

38 **Many other diseases:** Walter A. Orenstein and Rafi Ahmed, "Simply Put: Vaccination Saves Lives," *Proceedings of the National Academy of Sciences* 114, no. 16 (April 2017): 4031–33.

38 **In 2025, there has been:** Bhanvi Satija, "Measles Cases in Texas, New Mexico Rise to 294 as Outbreak Spreads," Reuters, March 14, 2025, sec. Healthcare & Pharmaceuticals.

38 **3 deaths and counting:** Neha Mukherjee and Deidre McPhillips, "Three Months into 2025, US Measles Cases Surpass Total for 2024," CNNHealth, March 14, 2025; "Texas Announces First Death in Measles Outbreak," Texas DSHS.

38 **The child who died:** Tom Bartlett, "His Daughter Was America's First Measles Death in a Decade," *The Atlantic*, March 11, 2025.

39 **Table 1: Deaths from:** *Pertussis (whopping cough):* "Pertussis Surveillance and Trends," CDC: Whooping Cough (Pertussis), January 13, 2025. *Diphtheria:* "Diphtheria Surveillance and Trends," CDC: Diphtheria, November

13, 2024. *Measles*: "Measles Cases and Outbreaks," CDC: Measles (Rubeola), accessed March 14, 2025; "Texas Announces First Death in Measles Outbreak," Texas Health and Human Services, Texas Department of State Health Services, February 26, 2025. *Rabies*: "Rabies in the United States: Protecting Public Health," CDC: Rabies, July 31, 2024. *Tetanus:* "Chapter 16: Tetanus," CDC: Manual for the Surveillance of Vaccine-Preventable Diseases, October 22, 2024. *Chickenpox:* "Chickenpox Vaccine Saves Lives Infographic," CDC: Chickenpox (Varicella), May 9, 2024. *Hepatitis B*: "Numbers and Rates of Deaths with Hepatitis B Virus Infections Listed as a Cause of Death Among Residents, by Demographic Characteristics—United States, 2017–2021," Table 2.8, CDC: Viral Hepatitis Surveillance, August 7, 2023. *Meningococcus:* "Meningococcal Disease Surveillance and Trends," CDC: Meningococcal Disease, November 12, 2024. *Rubella:* "Impact of U.S. MMR Vaccination Program. Rubella Elimination: A Public Health Success Story," CDC, January 17, 2025.

39 **Data indicate that people:** Maxime Taquet et al., "The Recombinant Shingles Vaccine Is Associated with Lower Risk of Dementia," *Nature Medicine* 30, no. 10 (October 2024): 2777–81.

40 **The lifetime risk of dying:** "Preventable Deaths: Odds of Dying," National Safety Council Injury Facts, accessed March 14, 2025.

40 **At that time, the highest:** Tom Kertscher, "Reports to the CDC's Vaccine Early Warning System Are Not 'Vaccine Deaths,'" PolitiFact, July 28, 2021.

40 **But by the end of July 2021:** "Covid: Fauci Says US Heading in Wrong Direction as Cases Rise," BBC, July 25, 2021.

40 **And among unvaccinated seniors:** "COVID-19 Hospitalizations and Deaths by Vaccination Status in Washington State," Washington State Department of Health, December 12, 2023.

40 **Another meta-analysis published:** Anderson E. Ikeokwu et al., "Unveiling the Impact of COVID-19 Vaccines: A Meta-Analysis of Survival Rates Among Patients in the United States Based on Vaccination Status," *Cureus* 15, no. 8 (August 2023); Andrew J. Shattock et al., "Contribution of Vaccination to Improved Survival and Health: Modelling 50 Years of the Expanded Programme on Immunization," *The Lancet* 403, no. 10441 (May 2024): 2307–16.

41 **To provide a comparison:** Michael M. McNeil and Frank DeStefano, "Vaccine-Associated Hypersensitivity," *Journal of Allergy and Clinical Immunology* 141, no. 2 (February 2018): 463–72.

41 **Meanwhile, out of the 2%:** J. Jiang et al., "Updated Pediatric Peanut Allergy Prevalence in the United States," *Annals of Allergy, Asthma & Immunology* 121, no. 5, S14, Supplement (November 2018); Jay A. Lieberman et al., "The Global Burden of Illness of Peanut Allergy: A Comprehensive Literature Review," *Allergy* 76, no. 5 (May 2021): 1367–84.

41 **nearly 3% of them:** Antonella Muraro et al., "Incidence of Anaphylaxis and Accidental Peanut Exposure: A Systematic Review," *Clinical and Translational Allergy* 11, no. 8 (October 2021): e12064.

41 **Unfortunately, in recent years:** Kevin Kuzminski, "U.S. Adults Are Still Behind on Routine Cancer Screenings—But Reasons Why Vary by Race," Prevent Cancer Foundation, April 1, 2024.

41 **For instance, according to the American Cancer Society:** Jessica Star et al., "Cancer Screening in the United States During the Second Year of the

COVID-19 Pandemic," *Journal of Clinical Oncology* 41, no. 27 (September 2023): 4352–59.

41 **up-to-date on cervical cancer screening:** "Cervical Cancer Screening," Cancer Trends Progress Report, National Cancer Institute, NIH, DHHS, Bethesda, MD, April 2025.

41 **One survey in 2024:** "U.S. Adults Are Still Behind on Routine Cancer Screenings," Prevent Cancer Foundation.

42 **For instance, there is a lot:** Uri Ladabaum et al., "Strategies for Colorectal Cancer Screening," *Gastroenterology* 158, no. 2 (January 2020): 418–32.

42 **Most of the US colorectal cancer deaths:** Reinier G. S. Meester et al., "Colorectal Cancer Deaths Attributable to Nonuse of Screening in the United States," *Annals of Epidemiology*, Causes of Cancer, 25, no. 3 (March 2015): 208–13.

42 **According to a 2022 landmark randomized-controlled trial:** Michael Bretthauer et al., "Effect of Colonoscopy Screening on Risks of Colorectal Cancer and Related Death," *New England Journal of Medicine* 387, no. 17 (October 2022): 1547–56; Angus Chen, "In Gold-Standard Trial, Invitation to Colonoscopy Reduced Cancer Incidence but Not Death," STAT, October 9, 2022.

42 **The good news:** "Why Is Colorectal Cancer Rising Rapidly Among Young Adults?," *Cancer Currents* (blog), National Cancer Institute, November 5, 2020.

42 **If you are between 50 and 80:** US Preventive Services Task Force et al., "Screening for Lung Cancer: US Preventive Services Task Force Recommendation Statement," *JAMA* 325, no. 10 (March 2021): 962.

42 **Through early detection:** US Preventive Services Task Force et al., "Screening for Lung Cancer."

43 **There is no scientific debate:** Roni Caryn Rabin, "When Should Women Get Regular Mammograms? At 40, U.S. Panel Now Says," *New York Times*, May 9, 2023, sec. Health; Barron H. Lerner, "Why Isn't There Agreement on When Women Need to Start Getting Mammograms?," STAT, May 2, 2024.

43 **In April 2024:** US Preventive Services Task Force et al., "Screening for Breast Cancer: US Preventive Services Task Force Recommendation Statement," *JAMA* 331, no. 22 (June 2024): 1918.

43 **The chance of a screening:** R. Edward Hendrick and Mark A. Helvie, "Mammography Screening: A New Estimate of Number Needed to Screen to Prevent One Breast Cancer Death," *American Journal of Roentgenology* 198, no. 3 (March 2012): 723–28.

43 **Finding cancer in women aged 50:** Hendrick and Helvie, "Mammography Screening."

43 **However, false positives:** Diana L. Miglioretti et al., "Association Between False-Positive Results and Return to Screening Mammography in the Breast Cancer Surveillance Consortium Cohort," *Annals of Internal Medicine* 177, no. 10 (October 2024): 1297–1307.

43 **But we do know:** "Cancer of the Breast (Female)—Cancer Stat Facts," SEER, accessed March 19, 2025.

43 **But only 61% of teens:** Melissa Jenco and News Content Editor, "HPV Vaccination Rate Stalls Again; 61% of Adolescents up to Date," *American Academy of Pediatrics Publications*, August 22, 2024; Cassandra Pingali,

"National Vaccination Coverage Among Adolescents Aged 13–17 Years—National Immunization Survey-Teen, United States, 2023," *MMWR Morbidity and Mortality Weekly Report* 73, (August 2024): 708–14.

43 **Further, nearly 25% of eligible women:** Ryan Suk et al., "Assessment of US Preventive Services Task Force Guideline—Concordant Cervical Cancer Screening Rates and Reasons for Underscreening by Age, Race and Ethnicity, Sexual Orientation, Rurality, and Insurance, 2005 to 2019," *JAMA Network Open* 5, no. 1 (January 2022): e2143582.

43 **The result is that over:** "Key Statistics for Cervical Cancer," American Cancer Society, January 16, 2025, accessed March 19, 2025; "Cervical Cancer," World Health Organization, March 5, 2024, accessed March 19, 2025.

44 **Between the ages of 20 and 29:** "Draft Recommendation Statement: Cervical Cancer: Screening," US Preventive Services Task Force, December 10, 2024, accessed March 19, 2025.

45 **The average age of diagnosis:** "Key Statistics for Prostate Cancer," American Cancer Society, May 30, 2025.

45 **That means that the vast majority:** C. Jacklin et al., "'More Men Die with Prostate Cancer Than Because of It'—An Old Adage That Still Holds True in the 21st Century," *Cancer Treatment and Research Communications* 26 (2021): 100225; "Survival Rates for Prostate Cancer," American Cancer Society, last modified November 22, 2023, accessed March 19, 2025.

45 **in studies that have used PSA testing:** Richard M. Martin, Emma L. Turner, Grace J. Young, et al., "Prostate-Specific Antigen Screening and 15-Year Prostate Cancer Mortality: A Secondary Analysis of the CAP Randomized Clinical Trial," *JAMA* 331, no. 17 (April 9, 2024): 1460–70; Jonas Hugosson, Monique J. Roobol, Marianne Månsson, Teuvo L. J. Tammela, Marco Zappa, et al., "A 16-yr Follow-Up of the European Randomized Study of Screening for Prostate Cancer," *European Urology* 76, no. 1(February 2019): 43–51.

45 **"the absolute mortality benefit was small":** Richard M. Martin et al.,"Prostate-Specific Antigen Screening."

46 **"[I]ndividuals at high risk":** H. Gilbert Welch and Tanujit Dey, "Testing Whether Cancer Screening Saves Lives: Implications for Randomized Clinical Trials of Multicancer Screening," *JAMA Internal Medicine* 183, no. 11 (August 2023): 1255–58.

46 **PSA testing reached a peak:** "Prostate Cancer Screening Trends Progress Report," National Cancer Institute, NIH, DHHS, Bethesda, MD, March 2024, accessed March 19, 2025.

46 **In 2012, USPSTF:** "Prostate Cancer: Screening (Archived)," US Preventive Services Taskforce, May 15, 2012, accessed March 19, 2025.

46 **Then in 2018:** US Preventive Services Task Force et al., "Screening for Prostate Cancer: US Preventive Services Task Force Recommendation Statement," *JAMA* 319, no. 18 (May 2018): 1901.

46 **Men who have a value:** "Tests to Diagnose and Stage Prostate Cancer," American Cancer Society, March 21, 2025, accessed March 19, 2025; Arihant Mehta et al., "Erectile Function Post Prostate Biopsy: A Systematic Review and Meta-Analysis," *Urology* 155 (September 2021): 1–8.

47 **"It [is] impossible to ignore":** "Behind the Headlines: PSA Screening Reduces Prostate Cancer Deaths but Can Miss Aggressive Cancer," Prostate Cancer UK, April 5, 2024.

48 **There are other screening tests:** US Preventive Services Task Force et al., "Screening for Hepatitis C Virus Infection in Adolescents and Adults: US Preventive Services Task Force Recommendation Statement," *JAMA* 323, no. 10 (March 2020): 970; US Preventive Services Task Force et al., "Screening for HIV Infection: US Preventive Services Task Force Recommendation Statement," *JAMA* 321, no. 23 (June 2019): 2326.

49 **A study of over 18 million:** David M. Studdert et al., "Homicide Deaths Among Adult Cohabitants of Handgun Owners in California, 2004 to 2016: A Cohort Study," *Annals of Internal Medicine* 175, no. 6 (June 2022): 804–11.

49 **The data on gun deaths:** John Gramlich, "What the Data Says About Gun Deaths in the U.S.," Pew Research Center, March 5, 2025.

49 **What's more, there are more gun deaths:** "All injuries," FastStats Homepage, CDC: National Center for Health Statistics, last modified July 23, 2024.

49 **Even more depressing:** Norah W. Friar et al., "Firearm Storage Behaviors— Behavioral Risk Factor Surveillance System, Eight States, 2021–2022," *MMWR. Morbidity and Mortality Weekly Report* 73, no. 23 (June 2024): 523–28.

49 **Irresponsibly stored and poorly maintained:** Jason E. Goldstick, Rebecca M. Cunningham, and Patrick M. Carter, "Current Causes of Death in Children and Adolescents in the United States," *New England Journal of Medicine* 386, no. 20 (May 2022): 1955–56.

49 **There are plenty:** "Newly Released Estimates Show Traffic Fatalities Reached a 16-Year High in 2021," National Highway Traffic Safety Administration, US Department of Transportation, May 17, 2022, accessed March 19, 2025.

49 **Think opioids:** "U.S. Overdose Deaths In 2021 Increased Half as Much as in 2020—But Are Still Up 15%," NCHS Pressroom, CDC: National Center for Health Statistics, last modified May 11, 2022; "Underlying Cause of Death, 2018–2023, Single Race Results Form," CDC WONDER, accessed March 19, 2025.

49 **There is no scientific evidence:** Ruben D. Acosta and Brooks D. Cash, "Clinical Effects of Colonic Cleansing for General Health Promotion: A Systematic Review," *American Journal of Gastroenterology* 104, no. 11 (October 2009): 2830–36.

50 **Moreover, cleansing has real risks:** "Why You Should Avoid Colon Cleansing," Cleveland Clinic Health Essentials, June 13, 2025; "Can Colon Cleansing Get Rid of Toxins from the Body?," Mayo Clinic, May 2024.

50 **And most bodies:** "Everest Dead Bodies: How Many People Have Died on Mount Everest?," Climbing Kilimanjaro, January 31, 2023.

50 **The older you are:** Raymond B. Huey et al., "Mountaineers on Mount Everest: Effects of Age, Sex, Experience, and Crowding on Rates of Success and Death," ed. Tim A. Mousseau, *PLOS ONE* 15, no. 8 (August 2020): e0236919.

50 **The inflection point:** Huey et al., "Mountaineers."

50 **"While summit success rates":** "The Bodies on Mount Everest: Dead, Frozen & Left at the Top," Ultimate Kilimanjaro, accessed June 6, 2024.

50 **These risks are way higher:** "Risk of Dying and Sporting Activities," *Bandolier*, archive.today webpage capture, last modified September 4, 2012.

50 **The injury rate in BASE:** Kjetil Soreide, Christian Lycke Ellingsen, and Vibeke Knutson, "How Dangerous Is BASE Jumping? An Analysis of

Adverse Events in 20,850 Jumps from the Kjerag Massif, Norway," *Journal of Trauma: Injury, Infection, and Critical Care* 62, no. 5 (May 2007): 1113–17.

50　**But skydiving might be:** Oliver Waite et al., "Sudden Cardiac Death in Marathons: A Systematic Review," *Physician and Sportsmedicine* 44, no. 1 (January 2016): 79–84.

Chapter 2: Talk to People

53　**At 92, he died peacefully:** Ezekiel J. Emanuel, "My 92-Year-Old Father Didn't Need More Medical Care," *The Atlantic*, January 2, 2020.

54　**My parents were the paradigmatic:** "Politics by Aristotle," trans. Benjamin Jowett, The Internet Classics Archive, MIT Classics, last modified 2009, accessed March 10, 2025. Ezekiel J. Emanuel, *Brothers Emanuel: A Memoir of an American Family* (Random House, 2013).

54　**Nearly 2,500 years ago, Aristotle:** "Nicomachean Ethics by Aristotle," trans. W. D. Ross, The Internet Classics Archive, MIT Classics, last modified 2009, accessed March 19, 2025.

55　**"June 29th. I gotta get in shape":** Paul Schrader, *Taxi Driver*, directed by Martin Scorsese (1976, Columbia Pictures).

55　**Or remember Alan Sillitoe's:** Alan Sillitoe, *The Loneliness of the Long-Distance Runner*, Harper Perennial Modern Classics ed. (Harper Perennial, 2007); Alan Sillitoe, *The Loneliness of the Long Distance Runner*, directed by Tony Richardson (1962, British Lion Films).

55　**"self-sufficent loners":** Ruchira Sharma, "Sigma Grindset: TikTok's Toxic Worshipping of Patrick Bateman Is Another Sign Young Men Are Lost," *British GQ*, November 7, 2022.

56　**The best and most interesting data:** "Second Generation Study," Harvard Study of Adult Development, Harvard Medical School, accessed March 19, 2025.

56　**The study enrolled:** Liz Mineo, "Good Genes Are Nice, but Joy Is Better," *Harvard Gazette*, April 11, 2017, sec. Health.

56　**Simultaneously, a Harvard criminology professor:** "Author Talks: The World's Longest Study of Adult Development Finds the Key to Happy Living," McKinsey & Company, February 16, 2023; Sheldon Glueck and Eleanor Glueck, *Unravelling Juvenile Delinquency* (Harvard University Press, 1950).

56　**While the two studies began separately:** Robert Waldinger and Marc Schulz, "What the Longest Study on Human Happiness Found Is the Key to a Good Life," *The Atlantic*, January 19, 2023.

56　**Today, these data:** "Second Generation Study," Harvard Medical School.

57　**Every 5 to 10 years, the men:** "Data Collection," Grant and Glueck studies, Adult Development Study, Harvard Medical School, accessed March 19, 2025.

57　**With about 85 years:** Waldinger and Schulz, "What the Longest Study on Human Happiness Found."

57　**"The people who were happiest":** "Author Talks," McKinsey & Company.

57　**"One crucial factor":** Robert Waldinger and Marc Schulz, *The Good Life: Lessons from the World's Longest Scientific Study of Happiness; Create a More Meaningful and Satisfying Life* (Simon & Schuster, 2023).

57　**There are many other long-term:** Julianne Holt-Lunstad, Timothy B. Smith, and J. Bradley Layton, "Social Relationships and Mortality Risk: A Meta-Analytic Review," ed. Carol Brayne, *PLOS Medicine* 7, no. 7 (July 2010):

e1000316; Craig A. Olsson et al., "A 32-Year Longitudinal Study of Child and Adolescent Pathways to Well-Being in Adulthood," *Journal of Happiness Studies* 14, no. 3 (June 2013): 1069–83.

58 **One of the biggest studies:** Yi Zeng, "Towards Deeper Research and Better Policy for Healthy Aging—Using the Unique Data of Chinese Longitudinal Healthy Longevity Survey," *China Economic Journal* 5, no. 2–3 (2012): 131–49.

58 **"to investigate the social":** Danan Gu et al., "Chinese Longitudinal Healthy Longevity Survey (CLHLS)," in *Encyclopedia of Gerontology and Population Aging*, ed. Danan Gu and Matthew E. Dupre (Springer International Publishing, 2021), 957–70.

58 **Between 1998 and 2018:** "Chinese Longitudinal Healthy Longevity Survey," Duke University Population Research Institute, Duke University, accessed March 20, 2025.

58 **For instance, playing cards:** Yaqi Li et al., "Social Isolation and Likelihood of Becoming Centenarians: Evidence from the Chinese Longitudinal Healthy Longevity Survey," *BMC Geriatrics* 24, no. 1 (October 2024): 839.

58 **Interestingly, they also found:** Li et al., "Social Isolation."

58 **Most importantly, while socializing monthly:** Ziqiong Wang et al., "Association Between Social Activity Frequency and Overall Survival in Older People: Results from the Chinese Longitudinal Healthy Longevity Survey (CLHLS)," *Journal of Epidemiology and Community Health* 77, no. 5 (May 2023): 277–84.

58 **Another piece of evidence:** "Welcome! Health and Retirement Study," Institute for Social Research, University of Michigan, accessed March 20, 2025.

58 **With repeated interviews:** E. S. Kim et al., "United We Thrive: Friendship and Subsequent Physical, Behavioural and Psychosocial Health in Older Adults (an Outcome-Wide Longitudinal Approach)," *Epidemiology and Psychiatric Sciences* 32 (2023): e65.

59 **Even after controlling for known risk:** Kristina Orth-Gomér and Jeffrey V. Johnson, "Social Network Interaction and Mortality," *Journal of Chronic Diseases* 40, no. 10 (January 1987): 949–57.

59 **Similarly, a more recent Australian study:** L. C Giles, "Effect of Social Networks on 10 Year Survival in Very Old Australians: The Australian Longitudinal Study of Aging," *Journal of Epidemiology & Community Health* 59, no. 7 (July 2005): 574–79.

59 **Much of the data:** Office of the Surgeon General (OSG), *Our Epidemic of Loneliness and Isolation: The U.S. Surgeon General's Advisory on the Healing Effects of Social Connection and Community* (US Department of Health and Human Services, 2023).

59 **"among initially healthy people":** Holt-Lunstad, Smith, and Layton, "Social Relationships and Mortality Risk."

59 **In fact, loneliness:** Holt-Lunstad, Smith, and Layton, "Social Relationships and Mortality Risk"; "Lacking social connection is comparable to smoking up to 15 cigarettes a day: FAQs," Resources, Julianne Holt-Lunstad, PhD, accessed March 20, 2025.

59 **Even more worrisome:** Julianne Holt-Lunstad et al., "Loneliness and Social Isolation as Risk Factors for Mortality: A Meta-Analytic Review," *Perspectives on Psychological Science* 10, no. 2 (March 2015): 227–37.

60 **Social connection has a profound:** Holt-Lunstad et al., "Loneliness and Social Isolation."

60 **Many studies have shown:** Sumathi Reddy, "How an Introvert Can Be Happier: Act Like an Extrovert," *Wall Street Journal*, July 23, 2013, sec. Health and Wellness.

60 **"Even highly introverted individuals":** Kiffer G. Card and Shayna Skakoon-Sparling, "Are Social Support, Loneliness, and Social Connection Differentially Associated with Happiness Across Levels of Introversion-Extraversion?," *Health Psychology Open* 10, no. 1 (January 2023).

60 **"misjudge how they will feel":** Reddy, "How an Introvert Can Be Happier."

60 **Researchers in Canada:** Anahita Shokrkon and Elena Nicoladis, "How Personality Traits of Neuroticism and Extroversion Predict the Effects of the COVID-19 on the Mental Health of Canadians," ed. Frantisek Sudzina, *PLOS ONE* 16, no. 5 (May 2021): e0251097.

60 **These long-term population studies:** Holt-Lunstad, Smith, and Layton, "Social Relationships and Mortality Risk."

61 **Researchers looked at people:** Chun Shen et al., "Plasma Proteomic Signatures of Social Isolation and Loneliness Associated with Morbidity and Mortality," *Nature Human Behaviour* 9 (January 2025): 569–83.

61 **In the longer term:** Shen et al., "Plasma Proteomic Signatures of Social Isolation."

62 **In 1990, 63% of Americans:** Daniel A. Cox, "The State of American Friendship: Change, Challenges, and Loss," Survey Center on American Life, AEI, June 8, 2021.

62 **As of 2015, that number:** Roberto A. Ferdman, "The Most American Thing There Is: Eating Alone," *Washington Post*, August 18, 2015, sec. Economic Policy; Laura Stampler, "Americans Eat More Than Half of Their Meals Alone," TIME, August 7, 2014, sec. Food & Drink.

62 **In 1984, the movie:** Ed. Weinberger and Stan Daniels, *The Lonely Guy*, directed by Arthur Hiller (1984, Universal Pictures).

62 **But responding to and encouraging:** Alissa Wilkinson, "The Glories of Dining Out Alone," *Vox*, January 26, 2023, sec. The Highlight; Lydia Swinscoe, "Why I Love Eating Alone in Restaurants," *Marie Claire*, October 24, 2023, sec. Travel.

62 **And it is worse among:** Jan-Emmanuel De Neve et al., "Sharing Meals with Others: How Sharing Meals Supports Happiness and Social Connections," Chapter 3: World Happiness Report, March 13, 2025.

62 **"The extent to which you share meals":** Sopan Deb, "Americans Are Unhappier Than Ever. Solo Dining May Be a Sign," *New York Times*, March 20, 2025, sec. U.S.

63 **People were bowling more:** Robert D. Putnam, *Bowling Alone: The Collapse and Revival of American Community* (Touchstone Books by Simon & Schuster, 2001).

63 **"deepening and intensifying":** Lulu Garcia-Navarro, "The Interview: Robert Putnam Knows Why You're Lonely," *New York Times*, July 13, 2024, sec. Magazine.

63 **"Social isolation increased":** Viji Diane Kannan and Peter J. Veazie, "US Trends in Social Isolation, Social Engagement, and Companionship—Nationally and by Age, Sex, Race/Ethnicity, Family Income, and Work Hours, 2003–2020," *SSM - Population Health* 21 (March 2023): 101331.

63 **Pew Research Center found:** Patrick van Kessel Smith, Chris Baronavski, Alissa Scheller, and Aaron Smith, "In Their Own Words, Americans Describe the Struggles and Silver Linings of the COVID-19 Pandemic," Pew Research Center, March 5, 2021.

63 **And younger Americans:** Jessica Buechler, "The Loneliness Epidemic Persists: A Post-Pandemic Look at the State of Loneliness among U.S. Adults," The Cigna Group, sec. News and Insights, accessed March 20, 2025.

66 **One of her characters:** Katie Hafner, *The Boys* (Spiegel & Grau, 2022).

66 **"'All you have to remember'":** Stav Atir, Xuan Zhao, and Margaret Echelbarger, "Talking to Strangers: Intention, Competence, and Opportunity," *Current Opinion in Psychology* 51 (June 2023): 101588.

66 **"One of the first times":** "Welcome," Gillian M. Sandstrom, accessed March 20, 2025.

67 **Enthralled by the transformative act:** Gillian M. Sandstrom and Erica J. Boothby, "Why Do People Avoid Talking to Strangers? A Mini Meta-Analysis of Predicted Fears and Actual Experiences Talking to a Stranger," *Self and Identity* 20, no. 1 (January 2021): 47–71.

67 **I was riding an Amtrak train:** Jonathan Eig, *King: A Life* (Farrar, Straus and Giroux, 2023).

68 **Gallup's World Poll:** Andrew Dugan, "Over 1 in 5 People Worldwide Feel Lonely a Lot," *Gallup*, July 10, 2024, sec. World.

68 **Some countries, such as Denmark:** Dugan, "Over 1 in 5 People Worldwide."

69 **By studying different primates:** R .I. M. Dunbar, "Neocortex Size as a Constraint on Group Size in Primates," *Journal of Human Evolution* 22, no. 6 (June 1992): 469–93.

69 **According to Dunbar:** Sheon Han, "You Can Only Maintain So Many Close Friendships," *The Atlantic*, May 20, 2021, sec. Family.

69 **Thus, 150 has become:** Dunbar, "Neocortex Size."

69 **Of these 150 people:** Han, "You Can Only Maintain So Many Close Friendships."

69 **But to transform that:** Jeffrey A. Hall, "How Many Hours Does It Take to Make a Friend?," *Journal of Social and Personal Relationships* 36, no. 4 (April 2019): 1278–96.

69 **It also requires:** Hall, "How Many Hours Does It Take to Make a Friend?"

71 **beginning at age 11:** Yunyu Xiao, Yuan Meng, Timothy T. Brown, et al.,"Addictive Screen Use Trajectories and Suicidal Behaviors, Suicidal Ideation, and Mental Health in US Youths," *JAMA* (online), June 18, 2025.

71 **A quarter of the teens:** Dimitri A. Christakis et al., "Adolescent Smartphone Use During School Hours," *JAMA Pediatrics* 179, no. 4 (February 2025): 475–78.

71 **Studies show that just seeing:** Jeanette Skowronek, Andreas Seifert, and Sven Lindberg, "The Mere Presence of a Smartphone Reduces Basal Attentional Performance," *Scientific Reports* 13, no. 1 (June 2023): 9363; Adrian F. Ward et al., "Brain Drain: The Mere Presence of One's Own Smartphone Reduces Available Cognitive Capacity," *Journal of the Association for Consumer Research* 2, no. 2 (April 2017): 140–54.

71 **"the mere presence of one's smartphone":** Ward et al., "Brain Drain."

72 **A recent study had participants:** Ryan J. Dwyer, Kostadin Kushlev, and Elizabeth W. Dunn, "Smartphone Use Undermines Enjoyment of Face-to-

Face Social Interactions," *Journal of Experimental Social Psychology* 78 (September 2018): 233–39.

72 **Though phones are marketed:** Dwyer, Kushlev, and Dunn, "Smartphone Use Undermines Enjoyment."

72 **If you are or plan to be:** Marcelo Toledo-Vargas, Kar Hau Chong, Claudia I. Maddren, et al., "Parental Technology Use in a Child's Presence and Health and Development in the Early Years: A Systematic Review and Meta-Analysis," *JAMA Pediatrics* (online), May 5, 2025.

73 **It certainly helps maintain:** Zach Rausch, Jonathan Haidt, and Lennon Torres, "Social-Media Companies' Worst Argument," *The Atlantic*, September 12, 2024, sec. Ideas.

74 **"participants who reported using":** Office of the Surgeon General (OSG), *Our Epidemic of Loneliness and Isolation: The U.S. Surgeon General's Advisory on the Healing Effects of Social Connection and Community, 2023* (US Department of Health and Human Services, 2023); Brian A. Primack et al., "Social Media Use and Perceived Social Isolation Among Young Adults in the U.S.," *American Journal of Preventive Medicine* 53, no. 1 (July 2017): 1–8.

74 **This is scary:** Jonathan Rothwell, "Teens Spend Average of 4.8 Hours on Social Media Per Day," *Gallup*, October 13, 2023, sec. Wellbeing.

74 **and nearly half:** Michelle Faverio and Olivia Sidoti, "Teens, Social Media and Technology 2024," Pew Research Center, December 12, 2024.

74 **One Italian study:** Valentina Rotondi, Luca Stanca, and Miriam Tomasuolo, "Connecting Alone: Smartphone Use, Quality of Social Interactions and Well-Being," *Journal of Economic Psychology* 63 (December 2017): 17–26.

74 **Over the last 2 decades:** "Speaking of Psychology: Why Our Attention Spans Are Shrinking, with Gloria Mark, PhD," American Psychological Association, accessed March 23, 2025; Gloria Mark, *Attention Span: A Groundbreaking Way to Restore Balance, Happiness and Productivity* (Hanover Square Press, 2023).

75 **"The use of social media may detract":** Louis Leung and Paul S. N. Lee, "Multiple Determinants of Life Quality: The Roles of Internet Activities, Use of New Media, Social Support, and Leisure Activities," *Telematics and Informatics* 22, no. 3 (August 2005): 161–80. Holly B. Shakya and Nicholas A. Christakis, "A New, More Rigorous Study Confirms: The More You Use Facebook, the Worse You Feel," *Harvard Business Review*, April 10, 2017, sec. Social Media; Dimitri A Christakis, "Internet Addiction: A 21st Century Epidemic?," *BMC Medicine* 8, no. 1 (December 2010): 61; Brian A. Feinstein et al., "Negative Social Comparison on Facebook and Depressive Symptoms: Rumination as a Mechanism," *Psychology of Popular Media Culture* 2, no. 3 (July 2013): 161–70.

75 **"was negatively associated":** Shakya and Christakis, "A New, More Rigorous Study Confirms"; Holly B. Shakya and Nicholas A. Christakis, "Association of Facebook Use with Compromised Well-Being: A Longitudinal Study," *American Journal of Epidemiology* 185, no. 3 (February 2017): 203–11.

75 **A recent study out of the United Kingdom:** Luisa Fassi, Amanda M. Ferguson, Andrew K. Przybylski, Tamsin J. Ford, and Amy Orben, "Social Media Use in Adolescents With and Without Mental Health Conditions," *Nature Human Behaviour* 9 (2025):1283–99.

75 **Getting off social media:** Jeffrey Lambert et al., "Taking a One-Week Break from Social Media Improves Well-Being, Depression, and Anxiety: A Randomized Controlled Trial," *Cyberpsychology, Behavior, and Social Networking* 25, no. 5 (May 2022): 287–93.

76 **Spending time in a park:** Mathew P. White et al., "Spending at Least 120 Minutes a Week in Nature Is Associated with Good Health and Wellbeing," *Scientific Reports* 9, no. 1 (June 2019): 7730.

76 **And a mountain of research shows:** Office of the Surgeon General (OSG), *Our Epidemic of Loneliness and Isolation*; Holt-Lunstad, Smith, and Layton, "Social Relationships and Mortality Risk"; Hamish M. E. Foster et al., "Social Connection and Mortality in UK Biobank: A Prospective Cohort Analysis," *BMC Medicine* 21, no. 1 (November 2023): 384; Lisa F. Berkman and S. Leonard Syme, "Social Networks, Host Resistance, and Mortality: A Nine-Year Follow-Up Study of Alameda County Residents," *American Journal of Epidemiology* 109, no. 2 (February 1979): 186–204.

76 **These are called "weak social ties":** Gillian M. Sandstrom and Elizabeth W. Dunn, "Social Interactions and Well-Being: The Surprising Power of Weak Ties," *Personality and Social Psychology Bulletin* 40, no. 7 (July 2014): 910–22.

77 **These mini-conversations:** Gillian M. Sandstrom and Elizabeth W. Dunn, "Is Efficiency Overrated?: Minimal Social Interactions Lead to Belonging and Positive Affect," *Social Psychological and Personality Science* 5, no. 4 (May 2014): 437–42.

77 **Another study of over 60,000:** Esra Ascigil et al., "Minimal Social Interactions and Life Satisfaction: The Role of Greeting, Thanking, and Conversing," *Social Psychological and Personality Science* 16, no. 2 (March 2025): 202–13.

77 **A different study showed:** Gul Gunaydin et al., "Minimal Social Interactions with Strangers Predict Greater Subjective Well-Being," *Journal of Happiness Studies* 22, no. 4 (April 2021): 1839–53.

77 **And a Japanese study found:** Itaru Ishiguro, "Minimal Social Interactions and Subjective Well-Being in the Japanese Context: Examination of Mediation Processes Using a National Representative Sample," *Social Sciences & Humanities Open* 8, no. 1 (October 2023): 100713.

77 **"[H]aving conversations with strangers":** Ascigil et al., "Minimal Social Interactions."

78 **A study in British workplaces:** William J. Fleming, "Employee Well-Being Outcomes from Individual-Level Mental Health Interventions: Cross-Sectional Evidence from the United Kingdom," *Industrial Relations Journal* 55, no. 2 (March 2024): 162–82.

78 **"Volunteering is the only type":** Fleming, "Employee Well-Being Outcomes."

78 **According to the researchers:** Fleming, "Employee Well-Being Outcomes."

78 **enhanced "social resources":** Fleming, "Employee Well-Being Outcomes."

79 **"Taking the steps":** Taylor Nicioli, "The Loneliness Epidemic: Nearly 1 in 4 Adults Feel Lonely, New Survey Finds," CNN Health, CNN, October 24, 2023.

Chapter 3: Expand Your Mind

80   **In 1776, at the ripe age:** Henry William Brands, *The First American: The Life and Times of Benjamin Franklin* (Anchor Books, 2002).

82   **He also noted the importance:** "Closing Speech at the Constitutional Convention (1787)," National Constitution Center, accessed March 21, 2025.

82   **Over 20,000 people attended:** Ezekiel J. Emanuel, "Benjamin Franklin and His World," Coursera, accessed March 21, 2025.

83   **"For having lived long":** "Closing Speech at the Constitutional Convention," National Constitution Center.

83   **Franklin is the paradigm:** Henry David Thoreau, *Walden* (Ticknor and Fields, 1854).

83   **Our brains literally shrink:** R. Peters, "Ageing and the Brain," *Postgraduate Medical Journal* 82, no. 964 (February 2006): 84–88.

84   *crystallized intelligence:* Raymond B. Cattell, "Theory of Fluid and Crystallized Intelligence: A Critical Experiment," *Journal of Educational Psychology* 54, no. 1 (February 1963): 1–22; Joshua K. Hartshorne and Laura T. Germine, "When Does Cognitive Functioning Peak? The Asynchronous Rise and Fall of Different Cognitive Abilities Across the Life Span," *Psychological Science* 26, no. 4 (April 2015): 433–43.

84   *fluid intelligence:* Cattell, "Theory of Fluid and Crystallized Intelligence"; Rogier A. Kievit et al., "The Neural Determinants of Age-Related Changes in Fluid Intelligence: A Pre-Registered, Longitudinal Analysis in UK Biobank," *Wellcome Open Research* 3 (June 2018): 38; Hartshorne and Germine, "When Does Cognitive Functioning Peak?"

84   **Working memory:** Lars Nyberg et al., "Memory Aging and Brain Maintenance," *Trends in Cognitive Sciences* 16, no. 5 (May 2012): 292–305.

85   **And they appear to decline:** Archana Singh-Manoux et al., "Timing of Onset of Cognitive Decline: Results from Whitehall II Prospective Cohort Study," *BMJ* 344 (January 2012); Laura Blue, "Study: Cognitive Decline Sets In as Early as Age 45," *Time,* January 6, 2012, sec. Aging, accessed March 21, 2025.

86   **There is a widespread theory:** C. Habeck et al., "Cognitive Reserve and Brain Maintenance: Orthogonal Concepts in Theory and Practice," *Cerebral Cortex* 27, no. 8 (August 2017): 3962–69.

86   **That first element:** Yaakov Stern, "What Is Cognitive Reserve? Theory and Research Application of the Reserve Concept," *Journal of the International Neuropsychological Society: JINS* 8, no. 3 (March 2002): 448–60.

86   **The second element:** Habeck et al., "Cognitive Reserve and Brain Maintenance."

87   **Researchers have noted:** Laura B. Zahodne et al., "The Role of Education in a Vascular Pathway to Episodic Memory: Brain Maintenance or Cognitive Reserve?," *Neurobiology of Aging* 84 (December 2019): 109–118; Jason Fletcher et al., "The Effects of Education on Cognition in Older Age: Evidence from Genotyped Siblings," *Social Science & Medicine* 280 (July 2021): 114044; Yuan S. Zhang et al., "Educational Attainment and Later-Life Cognitive Function in High- and Middle-Income Countries: Evidence from the Harmonized Cognitive Assessment Protocol," ed. Markus Schafer, *Journals of Gerontology, Series B: Psychological Sciences and Social Sciences* 79, no. 5 (May 2024): 1–12; Belén Guerra-Carrillo, Kiefer Katovich, and Silvia

A. Bunge, "Does Higher Education Hone Cognitive Functioning and Learning Efficacy? Findings from a Large and Diverse Sample," ed. Andrew R. Dalby, *PLOS ONE* 12, no. 8 (August 2017): e0182276; Xiangfei Meng and Carl D'Arcy, "Education and Dementia in the Context of the Cognitive Reserve Hypothesis: A Systematic Review with Meta-Analyses and Qualitative Analyses," *PLOS ONE* 7, no. 6 (2012): e38268.

88 **"A person with more education":** Martin Lövdén et al., "Education and Cognitive Functioning Across the Life Span," *Psychological Science in the Public Interest* 21, no. 1 (August 2020): 6–41.

88 **Yet, studies where researchers control:** K. A. Cagney and D. S. Lauderdale, "Education, Wealth, and Cognitive Function in Later Life," *Journals of Gerontology Series B: Psychological Sciences and Social Sciences* 57, no. 2 (March 2002): 163–72; D. Seblova, R. Berggren, and M. Lövdén, "Education and Age-Related Decline in Cognitive Performance: Systematic Review and Meta-Analysis of Longitudinal Cohort Studies," *Ageing Research Reviews* 58 (March 2020): 101005.

88 **While these brain connections:** Lövdén et al., "Education and Cognitive Functioning"; Nina Matyas et al., "Continuing Education for the Prevention of Mild Cognitive Impairment and Alzheimer's-Type Dementia: A Systematic Review and Overview of Systematic Reviews," *BMJ Open* 9, no. 7 (July 2019): e027719.

88 **"[I]t will take the individual":** Lövdén et al., "Education and Cognitive Functioning."

89 **Taking continuing education classes:** Matyas et al., "Continuing Education."

89 **Another proven method:** Peter Hudomiet, Michael D. Hurd, and Susann Rohwedder, "Identifying Early Predictors of Cognitive Impairment and Dementia in a Large Nationally Representative U.S. Sample," RAND, December 3, 2024, sec. Research.

89 **For example, learning a new language:** Giovanna Bubbico et al., "Effects of Second Language Learning on the Plastic Aging Brain: Functional Connectivity, Cognitive Decline, and Reorganization," *Frontiers in Neuroscience* 13 (May 2019): 423.

89 **or playing a musical instrument:** Sebastian Walsh, Robert Causer, and Carol Brayne, "Does Playing a Musical Instrument Reduce the Incidence of Cognitive Impairment and Dementia? A Systematic Review and Meta-Analysis," *Aging & Mental Health* 25, no. 4 (April 2021): 593–601; Ahmed Arafa et al., "Playing a Musical Instrument and the Risk of Dementia Among Older Adults: A Systematic Review and Meta-Analysis of Prospective Cohort Studies," *BMC Neurology* 22, no. 1 (October 2022): 395.

90 **Avoiding reckless behaviors:** Hudomiet, Hurd, and Rohwedder, "Identifying Early Predictors."

90 **They can cause chronic:** Harrison S. Martland, "Punch Drunk," *JAMA* 91, no. 15 (October 1928): 1103; Ann C. McKee et al., "The Neuropathology of Sport," *Acta Neuropathologica* 127, no.1 (January 2014): 29–51.

90 **"with longer careers not only were more likely":** Bobak Abdolmohammadi et al., "Duration of Ice Hockey Play and Chronic Traumatic Encephalopathy," *JAMA Network Open* 7, no. 12 (December 2024): e2449106.

90 **Not only have ultra-processed:** Melissa M. Lane et al., "Ultra-Processed Food Exposure and Adverse Health Outcomes: Umbrella Review of Epide-

miological Meta-Analyses," *BMJ Clinical Research Ed.* 384 (February 2024): e077310.

91 **The key finding:** Natalia Gomes Gonçalves et al., "Association Between Consumption of Ultraprocessed Foods and Cognitive Decline," *JAMA Neurology* 80, no. 2 (February 2023): 142.

91 **"a faster global cognition decline":** Gomes Gonçalves et al., "Association Between Consumption."

91 **On average, nearly 60%:** Julia A. Wolfson et al., "Trends in Adults' Intake of Un-Processed/Minimally Processed, and Ultra-Processed Foods at Home and Away from Home in the United States from 2003–2018," *Journal of Nutrition* 155, no. 1 (January 2025): 280–92; Filippa Juul et al., "Ultra-Processed Food Consumption Among US Adults from 2001 to 2018," *American Journal of Clinical Nutrition* 115, no. 1 (January 2022): 211–21.

91 **Nearly 70% of the calories:** Lu Wang et al., "Trends in Consumption of Ultraprocessed Foods Among US Youths Aged 2–19 Years, 1999–2018," *JAMA* 326, no. 6 (August 2021): 519.

91 **Indeed, the big food corporations:** Sarah Todd, "How Ultra-Processed Foods Captured the Baby and Toddler Market," STAT, February 26, 2025, sec. Health.

91 **"High UPF [ultra-processed food] intake":** Alex E. Henney et al., "High Intake of Ultra-Processed Food Is Associated with Dementia in Adults: A Systematic Review and Meta-Analysis of Observational Studies," *Journal of Neurology* 271, no. 1 (January 2024): 198–210.

91 **Though this connection is yet:** Jyri J. Virta et al., "Midlife Sleep Characteristics Associated with Late Life Cognitive Function," *Sleep* 36, no. 10 (October 2013): 1533–41; Xiao Tan et al., "Interactive Association Between Insomnia Symptoms and Sleep Duration for the Risk of Dementia—A Prospective Study in the Swedish National March Cohort," *Age and Ageing* 52, no. 9 (September 2023): 1–8; Séverine Sabia et al., "Association of Sleep Duration in Middle and Old Age with Incidence of Dementia," *Nature Communications* 12, no. 1 (April 2021): 2289; Shichan Wang et al., "Sleep Characteristics and Risk of Alzheimer's Disease: A Systematic Review and Meta-Analysis of Longitudinal Studies," *Journal of Neurology* 271, no. 7 (July 2024): 3782–93.

92 **Other studies have found:** Jayandra J. Himali et al., "Association Between Slow-Wave Sleep Loss and Incident Dementia," *JAMA Neurology* 80, no. 12 (December 2023): 1326.

92 **Some studies suggest:** Xuye Yuan et al., "Neural and Behavioral Evidence Supporting the Relationship Between Habitual Exercise and Working Memory Precision in Healthy Young Adults," *Frontiers in Neuroscience* 17 (April 2023); Paul D. Loprinzi et al., "Acute and Chronic Exercise Effects on Human Memory: What We Know and Where to Go from Here," *Journal of Clinical Medicine* 10, no. 21 (October 2021): 4812.

92 **In 2024, researchers at RAND:** Hudomiet, Hurd, and Rohwedder, "Identifying Early Predictors."

92 **The Whitehall II study:** M. G. Marmot et al., "Health Inequalities Among British Civil Servants: The Whitehall II Study," *The Lancet* 337, no. 8754 (June 1991): 1387–93.

92 **With interviews and cognitive tests:** Séverine Sabia et al., "Physical Activity, Cognitive Decline, and Risk of Dementia: 28 Year Follow-Up of Whitehall II Cohort Study," *BMJ* 357 (June 2017).

92 **It is a decline:** Sabia et al., "Physical Activity."

93 **The association between chronic disease:** Jessica G. Abell et al., "Association Between Systolic Blood Pressure and Dementia in the Whitehall II Cohort Study: Role of Age, Duration, and Threshold Used to Define Hypertension," *European Heart Journal* 39, no. 33 (September 2018): 3119–25.

93 **Individuals with 3 or more:** Céline Ben Hassen et al., "Association Between Age at Onset of Multimorbidity and Incidence of Dementia: 30 Year Follow-Up in Whitehall II Prospective Cohort Study," *BMJ* 376 (February 2022): e068005.

93 **"There is emerging consensus":** Singh-Manoux et al., "Timing of Onset of Cognitive Decline."

93 **"more frequent social contacts at age 60":** Andrew Sommerlad et al., "Association of Social Contact with Dementia and Cognition: 28-Year Follow-Up of the Whitehall II Cohort Study," *PLOS Medicine* 16, no. 8 (August 2019): e1002862.

94 **Or as two researchers argued:** Susann Rohwedder and Robert J. Willis, "Mental Retirement," *Journal of Economic Perspectives: A Journal of the American Economic Association* 24, no. 1 (2010): 119–38.

94 **Studies on retirement:** Ranu Sewdas et al., "Association Between Retirement and Mortality: Working Longer, Living Longer? A Systematic Review and Meta-Analysis," *Journal of Epidemiology and Community Health* 74, no. 5 (May 2020): 473–80; Sara Carmel and Aviad Tur-Sinai, "Cognitive Decline Among European Retirees: Impact of Early Retirement, Nation-Related and Personal Characteristics," *Ageing and Society* 42, no. 10 (October 2022): 2343–69; Annette Meng, Mette Andersen Nexø, and Vilhelm Borg, "The Impact of Retirement on Age Related Cognitive Decline—A Systematic Review," *BMC Geriatrics* 17, no. 1 (July 2017): 160; Raquel Fonseca, Arie Kapteyn, and Gema Zamarro, "Retirement and Cognitive Function," Pension Research Council, The Wharton School, University of Pennsylvania, 2016.

94 **"Five studies revealed":** Jessica Yauk, Britney Veal, and Debra Dobbs, "Understanding the Link Between Retirement Timing and Cognition: A Scoping Review," *Journal of Applied Gerontology* 43, no. 5 (May 2024): 588–600.

94 **My review of the data:** Sewdas et al., "Association Between Retirement and Mortality."

95 **In my view:** Rohwedder and Willis, "Mental Retirement."

95 **Indeed, countries like Belgium:** Rohwedder and Willis, "Mental Retirement."

95 **Thus, retiring at younger ages:** Rohwedder and Willis, "Mental Retirement."

95 **Similarly, this RAND study:** Hudomiet, Hurd, and Rohwedder, "Identifying Early Predictors."

96 **However, memory declined 38% faster:** Baowen Xue et al., "Effect of Retirement on Cognitive Function: The Whitehall II Cohort Study," *European Journal of Epidemiology* 33, no. 10 (October 2018): 989–1001.

96 **"long term detrimental effect":** Martina Celidoni, Chiara Dal Bianco, and Guglielmo Weber, "Retirement and Cognitive Decline: A Longitudinal Analysis Using SHARE Data," *Journal of Health Economics* 56 (December 2017): 113–25.

96 **A similar study from Norma Coe:** Norma B. Coe et al., "The Effect of Retirement on Cognitive Functioning," *Health Economics* 21, no. 8 (August 2012): 913–27.

97 **This may help resolve:** Celidoni, Dal Bianco, and Weber, "Retirement and Cognitive Decline."

97 **"it may be easier for some blue-collar workers":** Coe et al., "The Effect of Retirement on Cognitive Functioning."

98 **"When I met with a man":** "From Benjamin Franklin to Madame Brillon: Letter and Printed Bagatelle ('The Whistle'), 10 November 1779," Founders Online, National Archives, accessed April 16, 2025.

98 **"time for doing something useful":** Benjamin Franklin, *The Way to Wealth* (Applewood Books, 1986).

98 **"to read, study":** Benjamin Franklin, *Benjamin Franklin's Autobiography: A Norton Critical Edition*, ed. Joyce E. Chaplin (W. W. Norton, 2012).

Chapter 4: Eat Your Ice Cream

102 **Over 40% of adults:** "Overweight & Obesity Statistics," Health Statistics, NIH: National Institute of Diabetes and Digestive and Kidney Diseases (NIDDK), accessed January 25, 2024.

102 **Over 35% of American children:** "Overweight & Obesity Statistics," NIDDK.

102 **Projections show that:** Marie Ng et al.,"Global, Regional, and National Prevalence of Adult Overweight and Obesity, 1990–2021, with Forecasts to 2050: A Forecasting Study for the Global Burden of Disease Study 2021," *The Lancet* 405, no. 10481 (March 2025): 813–38.

102 **What we eat influences:** T. Ansari, N. S. Butt, and M. R. A. Hamid, "Effect of Diet on Type 2 Diabetes Mellitus: A Review," *International Journal of Health Sciences (Qassim)* 11, no. 2 (2017): 65–71; P. W. Lementowski and S. B. Zelicof, "Obesity and Osteoarthritis," *American Journal of Orthopedics* 37, no. 3 (2008): 148–51; Kunal Kulkarni et al., "Obesity and Osteoarthritis," *Maturitas* 89 (July 2016): 22–28.

102 **"healthier diets and lower":** Daria E. A. Jensen, et al., "Association of Diet and Waist-to-Hip Ratio With Brain Connectivity and Memory in Aging," *JAMA Network Open* 8, no. 3 (March 2025): e250171.

103 **Evolutionary biologists theorize:** T. Wu and S. Xu, "Understanding the Contemporary High Obesity Rate from an Evolutionary Genetic Perspective," *Hereditas* 160, no. 5 (February 2023).

103 **Indeed, applying the same criteria:** A. N. Gearhardt et al.,"Social, Clinical, and Policy Implications of Ultra-Processed Food Addiction," *BMJ* 383 (October 2023): e075354.

104 **By some measures:** J. E. Clapp et al.,"Changes in Serving Size, Calories, and Sodium Content in Processed Foods from 2009 to 2015," *Preventing Chronic Disease* 15 (March 2018): 170265.

104 **Consequently, average Americans:** "Once again, US and Europe Way Ahead on Daily Calorie Intake," UN News: Global Perspective Human Stories, United Nations, December 12, 2022, sec. Health.

104 **Americans consume 23%:** Drew Desilver, "What's on Your Table? How America's Diet Has Changed over the Decades," Pew Research Center, December 13, 2016.

104 **About half of all Americans:** "2024 IFIC Food & Health Survey," Food Insight, June 20, 2024.

104 **It can be frustrating:** Sripal Bangalore et al., "Body-Weight Fluctuations and Outcomes in Coronary Disease," *New England Journal of Medicine* 376 (April 2017): 1332–40.

104 **It is true that these drugs:** John P. H Wilding et al., "Once-Weekly Semaglutide in Adults with Overweight or Obesity," *New England Journal of Medicine* 384 (February 2021): 989–1002.

104 **And yes, this weight loss:** Michael A. Lincoff et al., "Semaglutide and Cardiovascular Outcomes in Obesity Without Diabetes," *New England Journal of Medicine* 389 (November 2023): 2221–32; Sunil V. Badve et al., "Effects of GLP-1 Receptor Agonists on Kidney and Cardiovascular Disease Outcomes: A Meta-Analysis of Randomized Controlled Trials," *The Lancet Diabetes & Endocrinology* 13, no. 1 (January 2025): 15–28; C. Y. Eren-Yazicioglu et al., "Can GLP-1 Be a Target for Reward System Related Disorders? A Qualitative Synthesis and Systematic Review Analysis of Studies on Palatable Food, Drugs of Abuse, and Alcohol," *Frontiers in Behavioral Neuroscience* 14 (January 2021): 614884.

105 **More importantly, after about a year:** D. H. Ryan et al., "Long-Term Weight Loss Effects of Semaglutide in Obesity Without Diabetes in the SELECT Trial," *Nature Medicine* 30 (May 2024): 2049–57.

105 **Most studies have found 12-month:** P. J. Rodriguez et al., "Discontinuation and Reinitiation of Dual-Labeled GLP-1 Receptor Agonists Among US Adults With Overweight or Obesity," *JAMA Network Open* 8, no. 1 (January 2025): e2457349.

105 **Losing weight then gaining it back:** Alison Z Swartz, Kathryn Wood, Eric Farber-Eger, Alexander Petty, and Heidi J Silver, "Weight Trajectory Impacts Risk for Ten Distinct Cardiometabolic Diseases, *Journal of Clinical Endocrinology & Metabolism,* June 11, 2025; Abigail Brooks, "Weight Cycling Increases Risk of MASLD, Other Cardiometabolic Diseases," HCP Live, June 18, 2025.

106 **Study after study shows:** Alec Tyson and Emma Kikuchi, "How Americans View Weight-Loss Drugs and Their Potential Impact on Obesity in the U.S," Pew Research Center, February 26, 2024; Kevin D. Hall and Scott Kahan, "Maintenance of Lost Weight and Long-Term Management of Obesity," *Medical Clinics of North America* 102, no. 1 (January 2018): 183–97; Susan A. Jebb and Paul Aveyard, "'Willpower' Is Not Enough: Time for a New Approach to Public Health Policy to Prevent Obesity," *BMC Medicine* 21, no. 89 (March 2023).

106 **Those 12-ounce cans of Coke:** "How Much Sugar Is Too Much?," Healthy Living, American Heart Association, last modified September 23, 2024, accessed March 21, 2025.

106 **No wonder that drinking:** Vasanti S. Malik et al., "Sugar-Sweetened Beverages and Risk of Metabolic Syndrome and Type 2 Diabetes: A Meta-Analysis," *Diabetes Care* 33, no. 11 (August 2010): 2477–83.

107 **Opting instead for the diet version:** Bee Wilson, "The Price of 'Sugar Free': Are Sweeteners as Harmless as We Thought?," *The Guardian,* December 8, 2022.

107 **But lots of research shows:** Wilson, "The Price of 'Sugar Free.'"

107 **Recently, WHO:** "WHO Advises Not to Use Non-Sugar Sweeteners for Weight Control in Newly Released Guideline," Departmental update, World Health Organization, May 15, 2023.

107 **Researchers at Israel's Weizmann Institute:** Jotham Suez et al., "Personalized Microbiome-Driven Effects of Non-Nutritive Sweeteners on Human Glucose Tolerance," *Cell* 185, no. 18 (September 2022): 3307–28.

109 **The peak year of soda:** "Per Capita Consumption of Soft Drinks in the United States from 2010 to 2018 (in Gallons)," Statista, May 1, 2019, accessed March 21, 2025.

109 **For instance, a recent report:** Y. Chen et al., "Consumption of Coffee and Tea with All-Cause and Cause-Specific Mortality: A Prospective Cohort Study," *BMC Medicine* 20, no. 449 (November 2022); T. Nguyen et al., "Coffee and Tea Consumption and the Risk of Head and Neck Cancer: An Updated Pooled Analysis in the International Head and Neck Cancer Epidemiology Consortium," *Cancer* 131, no. 2 (January 2025): e35620.

110 **Today, snacks contribute:** Ohio State University, "US Adults Eat a Meal's Worth of Calories of Snacks in a Day," ScienceDaily, December 15, 2023, accessed January 25, 2024.

110 **Indeed, the single largest source:** Sarah Rehkamp, "A Look at Calorie Sources in the American Diet," Amber Waves, United States Department of Agriculture Economic Research Service, December 5, 2016.

110 **Since 1970, Americans have consumed:** Desilver, "What's on Your Table?"

111 **For instance, General Mills sales:** Nathan Bomey, "The Snacking Recession: Why Americans Are Buying Fewer Treats," *Axios*, March 22, 2025, sec. Business.

112 **I focused my efforts:** Roxanne Roberts, "Breakfast Isn't a Sport. Zeke, One of the Emanuel Brothers, Would Beg to Differ," *Washington Post*, April 10, 2023.

113 **A recent review of 45 articles:** Megan M. Lane et al., "Ultra-Processed Food Exposure and Adverse Health Outcomes: Umbrella Review of Epidemiological Meta-Analyses," *BMJ* 384 (January 2024): e077310.

113 **They found that people:** Hyunju Kim, Emily A. Hu, and Casey M. Rebholz, "Ultra-Processed Food Intake and Mortality in the USA: Results from the Third National Health and Nutrition Examination Survey (NHANES III, 1988–1994)," *Public Health Nutrition* 22, no. 10 (February 2019): 1777–85.

114 **People who ate:** Kevin D. Hall et al., "Ultra-Processed Diets Cause Excess Calorie Intake and Weight Gain: An Inpatient Randomized Control Trial of *Ad Libitum* Food Intake," *Cell Metabolism* 30 (July 2019): 67–77.

114 **One theory:** Marta Tristan Asensi et al., "Low-Grade Inflammation and Ultra-Processed Foods Consumption: A Review," *Nutrients* 15, no. 6 (March 2023): 1546.

114 **Another idea:** Kevin Whelan et al., "Ultra-Processed Foods and Food Additives in Gut Health and Disease," *Nature Reviews Gastroenterology & Hepatology* 21 (February 2024): 406–27.

114 **Indeed, almost 60%:** Jennifer E. Clapp et al., "Changes in Serving Size, Calories, and Sodium Content in Processed Foods from 2009 to 2015," *Preventing Chronic Disease* 15 (March 2018): E33.

114 **And it's worse:** Lu Wang et al., "Trends in Consumption of Ultraprocessed Foods Among US Youths Aged 2–19 Years, 1999–2018," *JAMA* 326, no. 6

(August 2021): 519–30; University of Cambridge, "Ultra-Processed Food Makes Up Almost Two-Thirds of Calorie Intake of UK Adolescents, Study Finds," ScienceDaily, July 17, 2024.

114 **All told, it is estimated:** Sarah Todd, "How Ultra-Processed Foods Captured the Baby and Toddler Market," STAT, February 26, 2025, sec. Health.

115 **A measly 3 cookies:** Pepperidgefarm.com, accessed 4/29/25.

116 **The average human gut:** "Can Gut Bacteria Improve Your Health?," Harvard Health Publishing, Harvard Medical School, September 18, 2023, sec. Staying Healthy.

117 **Gut bacteria appear to play:** Livia H. Morais, Henry L. Schreiber IV, and Sarkis K. Mazmanian, "The Gut Microbiota–Brain Axis in Behaviour and Brain Disorders," *Nature Reviews Microbiology* 19 (October 2020): 241–55.

117 **An imbalance of bacteria:** Rue Dai et al.,"The Impact of the Gut Microbiome, Environment, and Diet in Early-Onset Colorectal Cancer Development," *Cancers* 16, no.3 (February 2024): 676.

117 **Consequently, fermented foods:** Kaitlin Vogel, "Eating 3 Servings of Kimchi Daily Linked to Lower Risk of Obesity," Healthline, January 30, 2024, sec. Health News.

117 **"steadily increased microbiota diversity":** Hannah C. Wastyk et al., "Gut-Microbiota-Targeted Diets Modulate Human Immune Status," *Cell* 184, no. 16 (August 2021): 4137–53.

118 **On average, Dutch men:** Gavin Haines, "Why Are the Dutch So Tall?," BBC, August 24, 2020.

118 **Interestingly, the Dutch became:** Gert Stulp et al., "Does Natural Selection Favour Taller Stature Among the Tallest People on Earth?," *Proceedings of the Royal Society B: Biological Sciences* 282, no. 1806 (May 2015): 20150211.

118 **There has been a lot of speculation:** Haines, "Why Are the Dutch So Tall?"

118 **The Netherlands:** "Milk Consumption by Country 2025," World Population Review, accessed March 24, 2025.

118 **Denmark is number one:** "Milk Consumption by Country 2025," World Population Review.

118 **Yogurt seems to protect:** Melissa Anne Fernandez and André Marette, "Potential Health Benefits of Combining Yogurt and Fruits Based on Their Probiotic and Prebiotic Properties," *Advances in Nutrition* 8, no. 1 (January 2017): 155S–164S.

118 **In one Harvard study:** Dariush Mozaffarian et al., "Changes in Diet and Lifestyle and Long-Term Weight Gain in Women and Men," *New England Journal of Medicine* 364, no. 25 (June 2011): 2392–2404.

119 **"countries with the highest intakes of milk":** Walter C. Willett and David S. Ludwig, "Milk and Health," *New England Journal of Medicine* 382, no.7 (February 2020): 644–54.

120 **"high-dairy intake showed no":** Eva Kiesswetter et al., "Effects of Dairy Intake on Markers of Cardiometabolic Health in Adults: A Systematic Review with Network Meta-Analysis," *Advances in Nutrition* 14, no. 3 (May 2023): 438–50.

120 **Full-fat milk has more:** Arne Astrup, Nina Rica Wium Geiker, and Faidon Magkos, "Effects of Full-Fat and Fermented Dairy Products on Cardiometabolic Disease: Food Is More Than the Sum of Its Parts," *Advances in Nutrition* 10, no. 5 (September 2019): 924S-930S.

120 **Dairy fat is protective:** Astrup, Geiker, and Magkos, "Effects of Full-Fat and Fermented Dairy Products."

120 **Some social media influencers:** "Channel: 200 Grams of Protein," Fitness Knowledge, TikTok, accessed March 21, 2025.

121 **"Protein is becoming":** Jordan Michelman, "Smells Like Protein Spirit," *TASTE*, January 1, 2025.

121 **The recommendation from a myriad:** Kim Painter, "Protein: Are You Getting Enough?," WebMD, December 17, 2023, sec. Health & Cooking Guide.

121 **Two exceptions:** Painter, "Protein."

122 **Indeed, leucine:** Yehui Duan et al., "The Role of Leucine and Its Metabolites in Protein and Energy Metabolism," *Amino Acids* 48, no. 1 (January 2016): 41–51; Marcus Waskiw-Ford et al., "Leucine-Enriched Essential Amino Acids Improve Recovery from Post-Exercise Muscle Damage Independent of Increases in Integrated Myofibrillar Protein Synthesis in Young Men," *Nutrients* 12, no. 4 (April 2020):1061.

122 **And maybe most surprising:** Thomas Laeger et al., "Leucine Acts in the Brain to Suppress Food Intake but Does Not Function as a Physiological Signal of Low Dietary Protein," *American Journal of Physiology–Regulatory, Integrative and Comparative Physiology* 307, no. 3 (August 2014): R310–20.

123 **One set of recommendations:** M. Rondanelli et al., "Where to Find Leucine in Food and How to Feed Elderly with Sarcopenia in Order to Counteract Loss of Muscle Mass: Practical Advice," *Frontiers in Nutrition* 7 (January 2021): 622391.

123 **Others suggest 5 grams:** Sarah Hammaker, "Leucine's Role in Muscle Synthesis," *Dieticians on Demand* (blog), September 25, 2023.

123 **According to the Department of Agriculture:** Grace Hussain, "Meat Consumption in the U.S.: Is It Increasing or Decreasing?," *Sentient*, December 22, 2023.

123 **Countries with better health:** "Per Capita Consumption of Meat," Our World in Data, Food and Agriculture Organization of the United Nations, accessed July 4, 2022.

124 **They are associated with weight gain:** Maryam S. Farvid et al., "Consumption of Red Meat and Processed Meat and Cancer Incidence: A Systematic Review and Meta-Analysis of Prospective Studies," *European Journal of Epidemiology* 36, no. 9 (August 2021): 937–51.

126 **A recent study of about 1,500:** Siran Lai, Guiting Zhou, Yue Li, Yuling Zhang, Yue An, Fuyuan Deng, et al., "Association Between Dietary Fiber Intake and Stroke Among US Adults: From NHANES and Mendelian Randomization Analysis," *Stroke* 56, no. 7 (April 29, 2025); Scott Buzby, "High Dietary Fiber Intake May Reduce Likelihood of Stroke, Death," *Cardiology Today*, Healio, May 20, 2025.

127 **This has long since:** Staff writer, "Forty Years of Low-Fat Diets: A 'Failed Experiment,'" Harvard T. H. Chan School of Public Health, October 7, 2016, sec. Chronic Diseases.

128 **And those so-called fish oils:** Ge Chen et al., "Regular Use of Fish Oil Supplements and Course of Cardiovascular Diseases: Prospective Cohort Study," *BMJ Medicine* 3 (May 2024): e000451.

129 **Studies have shown:** S. Sieri et al., "Glycemic Index, Glycemic Load, and

Risk of Coronary Heart Disease: A Pan-European Cohort Study," *American Journal of Clinical Nutrition* 112, no. 3 (September 2020): 631–43.

130   **On average, Americans eat:** "Growing Potatoes in Florida," University of Florida Institute of Food and Agricultural Sciences (IFAS Extension), accessed January 25, 2024.

130   **In one of my favorite dietary studies:** Dariush Mozaffarian et al., "Changes in Diet and Lifestyle and Long-Term Weight Gain in Women and Men," *New England Journal of Medicine* 364, no. 25 (June 2011): 2392–2404.

131   **Indeed, more than 70%:** "Sodium in Your Diet," Nutrition Education Resources & Materials, US Food and Drug Administration, last modified March 5, 2024.

131   **"The healthiest soups":** Perrin Braun, "Canned Versus Homemade Soup: What Are the Pros and Cons?," InsideTracker, March 6, 2024.

131   **As the American Heart Association says:** "How Much Sodium Should I Eat per Day?," Healthy Living, American Heart Association, accessed March 21, 2025.

131   **But acquiescing to the heavy salt:** "Sodium in Your Diet," USFDA.

132   **510 milligrams of salt:** McDonald's Nutrition Calculator, accessed 4/29/25.

132   **1,360 milligrams of salt:** McDonald's Nutrition Calculator, accessed 4/29/25.

132   **the deluxe version has 1,700 milligrams:** Chick-fil-A, Nutrition & Allergens.

132   **2,280 milligrams of salt:** Raising Cane's Allergen and Nutrition Information, accessed 4/29/25.

132   **Recent research shows:** D. K. Gupta et al., "Effect of Dietary Sodium on Blood Pressure: A Crossover Trial," *JAMA* 330, no. 23 (November 2023): 2258–66.

132   **"The blood pressure–lowering effect":** Gupta et al., "Effect of Dietary Sodium on Blood Pressure."

132   **People "who said":** Rui Tang et al., "Self-Reported Frequency of Adding Salt to Food and Risk of Incident Chronic Kidney Disease," *JAMA Network Open* 6, no. 12 (December 2023): e2349930.

133   **Alcohol in particular:** "Alcohol Use and Cancer," Cancer Risk and Prevention, American Cancer Society, last modified January 29, 2025, accessed March 24, 2025.

133   **A small exception:** Michael J. Thun et al., "Alcohol Consumption and Mortality Among Middle-Aged and Elderly U.S. Adults," *New England Journal of Medicine* 337, no. 24 (December 1997): 1705–14.

133   **Indeed, a study of nearly 314,000:** Lingling Zheng et al., "Association Between Alcohol Consumption and Incidence of Dementia in Drinkers: Linear and Non-Linear Mendelian Randomization Analysis," *The Lancet* 76 (October 2024): 102810.

133   **"Our findings suggested":** Zheng et al., "Association Between Alcohol Consumption and Incidence of Dementia."

134   **But this is not because:** "Are Organic Foods Worth the Price?," Nutrition and Healthy Eating, Mayo Clinic, accessed January 19, 2024.

134   **"There isn't a concrete study":** "Are Organic Foods Really Healthier?

Two Pediatricians Break It Down," *Good Food Is Good Medicine* (blog), UC Davis Health, April 5, 2019.

134 **Exposure to pesticides:** Chander Shekhar et al., "A Systematic Review of Pesticide Exposure, Associated Risks, and Long-Term Human Health Impacts," *Toxicology Reports* 13 (December 2024): 101840.

134 **"Low-level chronic dietary exposure":** Jessica Gama, Bianca Neves, and Antonio Pereira, "Chronic Effects of Dietary Pesticides on the Gut Microbiome and Neurodevelopment," *Frontiers in Microbiology* 13 (June 2022).

134 **I have often wondered:** James A. King et al., "Incidence of Celiac Disease Is Increasing Over Time: A Systematic Review and Meta-Analysis," *American Journal of Gastroenterology* 115, no. 4 (April 2020): 507–25.

137 **But a recent article:** David Merritt Johns, "Nutrition Science's Most Preposterous Result," *The Atlantic*, April 13, 2023, sec. Health.

137 **Skeptics ask who funded:** Merritt Johns, "Nutrition Science's Most Preposterous Result."

137 **This was the research conclusion:** Merritt Johns, "Nutrition Science's Most Preposterous Result."

137 **An even more interesting finding:** Andres V. Ardisson Korat, "Dairy Products and Cardiometabolic Health Outcomes" (SPH thesis, Harvard T. H. Chan School of Public Health, 2018); Mu Chen et al., "Dairy Consumption and Risk of Type 2 Diabetes: 3 Cohorts of US Adults and an Updated Meta-Analysis," *BMC Medicine* 12, no. 215 (November 2014); Merritt Johns, "Nutrition Science's Most Preposterous Result."

137 **Indeed, "ice cream was":** Merritt Johns, "Nutrition Science's Most Preposterous Result"; Mark A. Pereira et al., "Dairy Consumption, Obesity, and the Insulin Resistance Syndrome in Young Adults: The CARDIA Study," *JAMA* 287, no. 16 (April 2002): 2081–89.

137 **One theory:** Jing Guo et al., "The Impact of Dairy Products in the Development of Type 2 Diabetes: Where Does the Evidence Stand in 2019?," *Advances in Nutrition* 10, no. 6 (November 2019): 1066–75.

138 **But you also need:** David Hilzenrath, "This News Might Ruin Your Appetite—And Summer," KFF Health News, May 20, 2025.

139 **Unfortunately, most people:** Maura Judkis, "Do Millennials Really Not Know How to Cook? With Technology, They Don't Really Have to," *Washington Post*, April 12, 2018, sec. Food.

140 **The Chinese term for companion/partner:** Jan-Emmanuel De Neve et al., "Sharing Meals with Others: How Sharing Meals Supports Happiness and Social Connections," Chapter 3: World Happiness Report, March 13, 2025.

140 **"a third of weekday evening meals":** Robin M. Dunbar, "Breaking Bread: The Functions of Social Eating," *Adaptive Human Behavior and Physiology* 3, no. 3 (March 2017): 198–211; "Social Eating Connects Communities," University of Oxford News and Events, March 16, 2017.

140 **More recently, in 2023:** De Neve et al., "Sharing Meals with Others."

140 **"feel happier and are more satisfied":** Dunbar, "Breaking Bread."

141 **The distinguished epidemiologist:** Karen Glanz et al., "Diet and Health Benefits Associated with In-Home Eating and Sharing Meals at Home: A Systematic Review," *International Journal of Environmental Research and Public Health* 18, no. 4 (February 2021): 1577.

141 **less "violent behavior":** Megan E. Harrison et al., "Systematic Review of

the Effects of Family Meal Frequency on Psychosocial Outcomes in Youth," *Canadian Family Physician* 61, no. 2 (February 2015): e96–e106.

141 **It also improves:** Harrison et al., "Systematic Review of the Effects of Family Meal Frequency."

142 **"is a dominant synchronizer":** Anna Palomar-Cros et al., "Dietary Circadian Rhythms and Cardiovascular Disease Risk in the Prospective NutriNet-Santé Cohort," *Nature Communications* 14, no 7899 (December 2023).

143 **Omitting breakfast is associated:** Richard Ofori-Asenso, Alice J. Owen, and Danny Liew, "Skipping Breakfast and the Risk of Cardiovascular Disease and Death: A Systematic Review of Prospective Cohort Studies in Primary Prevention Settings," *Journal of Cardiovascular Development and Disease* 6, no. 3 (August 2019): 30.

143 **Compared with eating breakfast:** Palomar-Cros et al., "Dietary Circadian Rhythms."

143 **Second, avoid late-night snacking:** Palomar-Cros et al., "Dietary Circadian Rhythms."

143 **For reducing the risk:** Palomar-Cros et al., "Dietary Circadian Rhythms."

143 **Finally, there is evidence:** Palomar-Cros et al., "Dietary Circadian Rhythms."

143 **These studies show that consuming:** Dae-Kyu Song and Yong-Woon Kim, "Beneficial Effects of Intermittent Fasting: A Narrative Review," *Journal of Yeungnam Medical Sciences* 40, no. 1 (April 2022): 4–11.

143 **These pathways also trigger:** Song and Kim, "Beneficial Effects of Intermittent Fasting."

144 **Some data suggest:** Satchin Panda, *The Circadian Diabetes Code* (Rodale, 2021).

144 **This worked for eating:** Panda, *The Circadian Diabetes Code.*

144 **fasting "slows or reverses aging":** Rafael de Cabo and Mark P. Mattson, "Effects of Intermittent Fasting on Health, Aging, and Disease," *New England Journal of Medicine* 381, no. 26 (December 2019): 2541–51.

144 **Subsequently, other researchers:** Deying Liu et al., "Calorie Restriction with or Without Time-Restricted Eating in Weight Loss," *New England Journal of Medicine* 386, no. 16 (April 2022): 1495–1504.

146 **As many as 75% of adult:** "CRN Reveals Survey Data from 2022 Consumer Survey on Dietary Supplements," Council for Responsible Nutrition, October 13, 2022, sec. Newsroom, accessed January 25, 2024.

146 **Unfortunately, thanks to Senator Orrin Hatch:** W. Steven Pray, "Orrin Hatch and the Dietary Supplement Health and Education Act: Pandora's Box Revisited," *Journal of Child Neurology* 27, no. 5 (May 2012): 561–63.

146 **Vitamins A and E:** Wei Qi Loh et al., "Association Between Vitamin A and E Forms and Prostate Cancer Risk in the Singapore Prostate Cancer Study," *Nutrients* 15, no. 12 (June 2023): 2677.

146 **So, too, does beta-carotene:** "Beta Carotene (Oral Route)," Drugs & Supplements, Mayo Clinic, accessed February 2, 2024.

146 **And some supplements:** João Guilherme Costa et al.,"Contaminants: A Dark Side of Food Supplements?," *Free Radical Research* 53, no. Suppl. 1 (September 2019): 1113–35.

147 **Americans spend about $12 billion:** "Is There Really Any Benefit to

Multivitamins?," Wellness and Prevention, Johns Hopkins Medicine, accessed March 22, 2025.

147 **The Physicians' Health Study II:** J. Michael Gaziano et al., "Multivitamins in the Prevention of Cancer in Men: The Physicians' Health Study II Randomized Controlled Trial," *JAMA* 308, no. 18 (November 2012): 1871–80.

147 **Data from a meta-analysis:** Stephen P. Fortmann et al., "Vitamin and Mineral Supplements in the Primary Prevention of Cardiovascular Disease and Cancer: An Updated Systematic Evidence Review for the U.S. Preventive Services Task Force," *Annals of Internal Medicine* 159, no. 12 (December 2013): 824–34.

147 **As a group of Johns Hopkins researchers:** Eliseo Guallar et al., "Enough Is Enough: Stop Wasting Money on Vitamin and Mineral Supplements," *Annals of Internal Medicine* 159, no. 12 (December 2013): 850–51.

148 **"elixir of life":** Parminder Singh, Kishore Gollapalli, Stefano Mangiola, Daniela Schranner, Vijay K. Yadav, et al., "Taurine Deficiency as a Driver of Aging," *Science* 380, no. 6649 (June 9, 2023); Sandee LaMotte, "Is Taurine the 'Elixir of Life'? Maybe, If You're a Worm, Mouse or Monkey," CNN Health, June 8, 2023.

148 **"On the basis of these findings":** Maria Emilia Fernandez, Michel Bernier, Nathan L. Price, Simonetta Camandola, Rafael de Cabo, et al., "Is Taurine an Aging Biomarker?," *Science* 388, no. 6751 (June 5, 2025).

Chapter 5: Move It!

151 **Indeed, my father's preferred exercise:** Dan Buettner, *The Blue Zones: Lessons for Living Longer from the People Who've Lived the Longest,* illustrated edition (National Geographic, 2010); Institute of Medicine Roundtable on Population Health Improvement, "Lessons from the Blue Zones®," in *Business Engagement in Building Healthy Communities: Workshop Summary* (National Academies Press, 2015).

152 **An assessment of nearly 32,000:** Christiaan G. Abildso et al., "Prevalence of Meeting Aerobic, Muscle-Strengthening, and Combined Physical Activity Guidelines During Leisure Time Among Adults, by Rural-Urban Classification and Region—United States, 2020," *MMWR. Morbidity and Mortality Weekly Report* 72, no. 4 (January 2023): 85–89.

152 **That means that 72%:** Abildso et al., "Prevalence of Meeting Aerobic, Muscle-Strengthening, and Combined Physical Activity Guidelines."

152 **Perhaps this is because 82%:** Charles E. Matthews et al., "Sedentary Behavior in U.S. Adults: Fall 2019," *Medicine & Science in Sports & Exercise* 53, no. 12 (December 2021): 2512–19.

152 **While a large majority:** "Adult Physical Inactivity Outside of Work," CDC: Physical Activity, January 31, 2025.

152 **Sedentary drivers:** Ding Ding and Ulf Ekelund, "From London Buses to Activity Trackers: A Reflection of 70 Years of Physical Activity Research," *Journal of Sport and Health Science* 13, no. 6 (November 2024): 736–38.

152 **This finding holds true:** J. N. Morris et al., "Coronary Heart-Disease and Physical Activity of Work," *The Lancet* 262, no. 6795 (November 1953): 1053–57; Ralph S. Paffenbarger, Jr., Steven N. Blair, and I-Min Lee, "A History of Physical Activity, Cardiovascular Health and Longevity: The Scientific Contributions of Jeremy N Morris, DSc, DPH, FRCP," *International Journal of Epidemiology* 30, no. 5 (October 2001): 1184–92.

153 **It reduces the risk:** "Physical Activity," World Health Organization, June 26, 2024, accessed March 25, 2025.

153 **It can also positively:** Kathleen Mikkelsen et al., "Exercise and Mental Health," *Maturitas* 106 (December 2017): 48–56; Elizabeth Anderson and Geetha Shivakumar, "Effects of Exercise and Physical Activity on Anxiety," *Frontiers in Psychiatry* 4 (April 2013): 27.

153 **people who are "insufficiently active":** "Physical Activity," World Health Organization.

153 **A meta-analysis:** Leandro Garcia et al., "Non-Occupational Physical Activity and Risk of Cardiovascular Disease, Cancer and Mortality Outcomes: A Dose–Response Meta-Analysis of Large Prospective Studies," *British Journal of Sports Medicine* 57, no. 15 (August 2023): 979–89.

153 **Exercising as little as 15 minutes:** Chi Pang Wen et al., "Minimum Amount of Physical Activity for Reduced Mortality and Extended Life Expectancy: A Prospective Cohort Study," *The Lancet* 378, no. 9798 (October 2011): 1244–53.

153 **In one study, researchers enrolled:** James A. Blumenthal et al., "Lifestyle and Neurocognition in Older Adults with Cognitive Impairments: A Randomized Trial," *Neurology* 92, no. 3 (January 2019): e212–e223.

154 **One year follow-up:** James A. Blumenthal et al., "Longer Term Effects of Diet and Exercise on Neurocognition: 1-Year Follow-Up of the ENLIGHTEN Trial," *Journal of the American Geriatrics Society* 68, no. 3 (March 2020): 559–68.

154 **Exercise also has the side benefit:** Katrina L. Piercy et al., "The Physical Activity Guidelines for Americans," *JAMA* 320, no. 19 (November 2018): 2020.

154 **Exercise is proven to:** Majd A. Alnawwar et al., "The Effect of Physical Activity on Sleep Quality and Sleep Disorder: A Systematic Review," *Cureus* 15, no. 8 (August 2023): e43595; M. Alexandra Kredlow et al., "The Effects of Physical Activity on Sleep: A Meta-Analytic Review," *Journal of Behavioral Medicine* 38, no. 3 (June 2015): 427–49; Hayley Lowe et al., "Does Exercise Improve Sleep for Adults with Insomnia? A Systematic Review with Quality Appraisal," *Clinical Psychology Review* 68 (March 2019): 1–12.

154 **"Virtually any form of exercise":** Mayo Clinic Staff, "Exercise and Stress: Get Moving to Manage Stress," Mayo Clinic, last modified March 26, 2025.

154 **Add some amount:** Steven N. Blair, "Physical Fitness and All-Cause Mortality: A Prospective Study of Healthy Men and Women," *JAMA* 262, no. 17 (November 1989): 2395.

155 **This strengthens the heart muscle:** Robert Ambrogetti, "The Effects of Exercise on Coronary Collateral Circulation: A Review," *Cureus* 14, no. 12 (December 2022): e32732; Sven Möbius-Winkler et al., "Coronary Collateral Growth Induced by Physical Exercise: Results of the Impact of Intensive Exercise Training on Coronary Collateral Circulation in Patients with Stable Coronary Artery Disease (EXCITE) Trial," *Circulation* 133, no. 15 (April 2016): 1438–48.

155 **This collateral flow:** Pascal Meier et al., "The Impact of the Coronary Collateral Circulation on Mortality: A Meta-Analysis," *European Heart Journal* 33, no. 5 (March 2012): 614–21; Jeroen Koerselman et al., "Coronary Collaterals: An Important and Underexposed Aspect of Coronary Artery Disease," *Circulation* 107, no. 19 (May 2003): 2507–11.

155 **Sustained exercise also improves:** Steven Mann, Christopher Beedie, and Alfonso Jimenez, "Differential Effects of Aerobic Exercise, Resistance Training and Combined Exercise Modalities on Cholesterol and the Lipid Profile: Review, Synthesis and Recommendations," *Sports Medicine (Auckland, N.Z.)* 44, no. 2 (February 2014): 211–21.

155 **It increases the uptake:** Jonathan M. Memme et al., "Exercise and Mitochondrial Health," *Journal of Physiology* 599, no. 3 (February 2021): 803–17; Ashley N. Oliveira and David A. Hood, "Exercise Is Mitochondrial Medicine for Muscle," *Sports Medicine and Health Science* 1, no. 1 (December 2019): 11–18.

155 **Exercise also increases the sensitivity:** Stephen R. Bird and John A. Hawley, "Update on the Effects of Physical Activity on Insulin Sensitivity in Humans," *BMJ Open Sport & Exercise Medicine* 2, no. 1 (March 2017): e000143; Tyler E. Keshel and Robert H. Coker, "Exercise Training and Insulin Resistance: A Current Review," *Journal of Obesity & Weight Loss Therapy* 5, no. Suppl. 5 (July 2015): S5–003; Maha Sellami et al., "Eight Weeks of Aerobic Exercise, but Not Four, Improves Insulin Sensitivity and Cardiovascular Performance in Young Women," *Scientific Reports* 15, no. 1 (January 2025): 1991.

155 **Finally, exercise places stress:** "Lactic Acid," Health Library, Cleveland Clinic, last modified December 9, 2022.

155 **A similar idea:** "Slowing Bone Loss with Weight-Bearing Exercise," Harvard Health Publishing, April 11, 2021, sec. Staying Healthy.

156 **Exercise and other weight-bearing:** Lívia Santos, Kirsty Jayne Elliott-Sale, and Craig Sale, "Exercise and Bone Health Across the Lifespan," *Biogerontology* 18, no. 6 (December 2017): 931–46.

156 **If you are 60:** "Target Heart Rates Chart," American Heart Association, last modified August 12, 2024, accessed March 25, 2025.

156 **So vigorous activity:** "Target Heart Rates Chart," American Heart Association.

157 **Instead, just use Table 6:** "Measuring Physical Activity Intensity," CDC: Physical Activity, last modified June 3, 2022.

157 **During vigorous-intensity activities:** "Measuring Physical Activity Intensity," CDC.

157 **Some researchers have postulated:** Alex Hutchinson, "Is 'Zone 2' the Magic Effort Level for Exercise?," *New York Times*, February 19, 2025, sec. Well.

158 **Given its alignment:** Ashwin Rodrigues, "Zone 2 Training: Why Long, Easy Workouts Became the Biggest Thing in Fitness," *GQ*, January 24, 2025, sec. Wellness.

158 **In fact, "per total hour":** Knut Sindre Mølmen, Nicki Winfield Almquist, and Øyvind Skattebo, "Effects of Exercise Training on Mitochondrial and Capillary Growth in Human Skeletal Muscle: A Systematic Review and Meta-Regression," *Sports Medicine* 55, no. 1 (January 2025): 115–44.

159 **Muscle mass only:** Elena Volpi, Reza Nazemi, and Satoshi Fujita, "Muscle Tissue Changes with Aging," *Current Opinion in Clinical Nutrition and Metabolic Care* 7, no. 4 (July 2004): 405–10.

159 **It really starts to plummet:** D. J. Wilkinson, M. Piasecki, and P. J. Atherton, "The Age-Related Loss of Skeletal Muscle Mass and Function: Measurement and Physiology of Muscle Fibre Atrophy and Muscle Fibre Loss in

Humans," *Ageing Research Reviews* 47 (November 2018): 123–32; "Age and Muscle Loss," Harvard Health Publishing, (February 14, 2023).

159 **"short-term muscle inactivity":** Volpi, Nazemi, and Fujita, "Muscle Tissue Changes with Aging."

159 **keeping people stronger:** Volpi, Nazemi, and Fujita, "Muscle Tissue Changes with Aging."

160 **It is more of a social game:** "2024 Adult Compendium," Compendium of Physical Activities, December 4, 2023.

160 **A comprehensive review:** Jack Luscombe et al., "A Rapid Review to Identify Physical Activity Accrued While Playing Golf," *BMJ Open* 7, no. 11 (November 2017): e018993.

161 **"golf *can* provide moderate intensity":** A. D. Murray et al., "The Relationships Between Golf and Health: A Scoping Review," *British Journal of Sports Medicine* 51, no. 1 (January 2017): 12–19; Luscombe et al., "A Rapid Review."

161 **"golfers may find it difficult":** Luscombe et al., "A Rapid Review."

161 **So, a weekly golf game:** "2024 Adult Compendium," Compendium of Physical Activities.

162 **Think woodpeckers:** Jenny McKee, "New Study Shakes Up Long-Held Belief on Woodpecker Hammering," *Audubon*, July 14, 2022, sec. News.

162 **A growing body of evidence:** Michael Saulle and Brian D. Greenwald, "Chronic Traumatic Encephalopathy: A Review," *Rehabilitation Research and Practice* 2012, no. 816069 (2012): 1–9.

162 **A chilling article:** Ann C. McKee et al., "Neuropathologic and Clinical Findings in Young Contact Sport Athletes Exposed to Repetitive Head Impacts," *JAMA Neurology* 80, no. 10 (October 2023): 1037.

162 **Among the 152 young athletes:** McKee et al., "Neuropathologic and Clinical Findings."

162 **Another recent study of 77:** Bobak Abdolmohammadi et al., "Duration of Ice Hockey Play and Chronic Traumatic Encephalopathy," *JAMA Network Open* 7, no. 12 (December 2024): e2449106.

162 **About 20% of players:** Abdolmohammadi et al., "Duration of Ice Hockey Play."

163 **The CDC recommends:** "Adult Activity: An Overview," CDC: Physical Activity Basics, December 20, 2023.

163 **A long-term, 30-year follow-up:** Dong Hoon Lee et al., "Long-Term Leisure-Time Physical Activity Intensity and All-Cause and Cause-Specific Mortality: A Prospective Cohort of US Adults," *Circulation* 146, no. 7 (August 2022): 523–34.

163 **Similarly, people doing 300 to 600:** Lee et al., "Long-Term Leisure-Time Physical Activity."

164 **Importantly, there didn't seem:** Lee et al., "Long-Term Leisure-Time Physical Activity."

165 **"helmets decrease the potential":** Daniel H. Daneshvar et al., "Helmets and Mouth Guards: The Role of Personal Equipment in Preventing Sport-Related Concussions," *Clinics in Sports Medicine* 30, no. 1 (January 2011): 145–63.

165 **A meta-analysis of 55 studies:** Alena Høye, "Bicycle Helmets—To Wear or Not to Wear? A Meta-Analyses of the Effects of Bicycle Helmets on Injuries," *Accident Analysis & Prevention* 117 (August 2018): 85–97.

165 **"there is moderate to strong evidence":** Katie Small, Lars McNaughton, and Martyn Matthews, "A Systematic Review into the Efficacy of Static

Stretching as Part of a Warm-Up for the Prevention of Exercise-Related Injury," *Research in Sports Medicine* 16, no. 3 (September 2008): 213–31.

165 **However, there is growing:** Small, McNaughton, and Matthews, "A Systematic Review into the Efficacy of Static Stretching"; Helmi Chaabene et al., "Acute Effects of Static Stretching on Muscle Strength and Power: An Attempt to Clarify Previous Caveats," *Frontiers in Physiology* 10 (November 2019): 1468.

165 **"The relationship between stretching":** José Afonso, Jesús Olivares-Jabalera, and Renato Andrade, "Time to Move from Mandatory Stretching? We Need to Differentiate 'Can I?' From 'Do I Have To?,'" *Frontiers in Physiology* 12 (July 2021): 714166.

166 **A recent review of 15 studies:** Liyi Ding et al., "Effectiveness of Warm-Up Intervention Programs to Prevent Sports Injuries Among Children and Adolescents: A Systematic Review and Meta-Analysis," *International Journal of Environmental Research and Public Health* 19, no. 10 (May 2022): 6336.

166 **There is even a name:** Rupert P. Williams et al., "'Warm-Up Angina': Harnessing the Benefits of Exercise and Myocardial Ischaemia," *Heart* 100, no. 2 (January 15, 2014): 106–14.

166 **This phenomenon:** Rupert P. Williams et al., "Republished: 'Warm-Up Angina': Harnessing the Benefits of Exercise and Myocardial Ischaemia," *Postgraduate Medical Journal* 90, no. 1069 (November 2014): 648–56.

167 **Research shows:** Scott B. Shawen, Theodora Dworak, and Robert B. Anderson, "Return to Play Following Ankle Sprain and Lateral Ligament Reconstruction," *Clinics in Sports Medicine* 35, no. 4 (October 2016): 697–709.

167 **One study showed:** Susanne Beischer et al., "Young Athletes Who Return to Sport Before 9 Months After Anterior Cruciate Ligament Reconstruction Have a Rate of New Injury 7 Times That of Those Who Delay Return," *Journal of Orthopaedic & Sports Physical Therapy* 50, no. 2 (February 2020): 83–90.

168 **A 19-year study:** William O. Roberts and Steven D. Stovitz, "Incidence of Sudden Cardiac Death in Minnesota High School Athletes 1993–2012 Screened with a Standardized Pre-Participation Evaluation," *Journal of the American College of Cardiology* 62, no. 14 (October 2013): 1298–1301.

168 **However, from the data:** Jonathan H. Kim, Austin J. Rim, James T. Miller, et al., "Cardiac Arrest During Long-Distance Running Races," *JAMA* 333, no. 19 (May 2025): 1699–1707.

169 **The cardiac advantages:** Knvul Sheikh, "How Long Does It Take to Get Fit Again?," *New York Times*, January 30, 2023, sec. Well.

169 **Just 2 months:** Sheikh, "How Long Does It Take to Get Fit Again?"

169 **And there are other changes:** Erin Carter, "The Effects of Stopping Exercise: Part One," MSU Extension, Michigan State University, November 9, 2016.

169 **Higher blood pressure:** Carter, "The Effects of Stopping Exercise."

170 **The absolute highest $\dot{V}O_2$ max:** Robert Wood, "VO_{2max} World Records," Topend Sports, accessed March 25, 2025.

170 **Results from a 2020 study:** James E. Peterman et al., "Development of Global Reference Standards for Directly Measured Cardiorespiratory Fitness: A Report from the Fitness Registry and Importance of Exercise National Database (FRIEND)," *Mayo Clinic Proceedings* 95, no. 2 (February 2020): 255–64.

170 **"VO₂ max is one of":** Dan E. Webster et al., "Smartphone-Based VO₂max Measurement with Heart Snapshot in Clinical and Real-World Settings with a Diverse Population: Validation Study," *JMIR mHealth and uHealth* 9, no. 6 (June 2021): e26006.

170 **Unfortunately, V̇O₂ max declines:** Peterman et al., "Development of Global Reference Standards."

171 **As a major study:** Darryl P. Leong et al., "Prognostic Value of Grip Strength: Findings from the Prospective Urban Rural Epidemiology (PURE) Study," *The Lancet* 386, no. 9990 (July 2015): 266–73.

171 **Instead, we do more:** Elizabeth Fain and Cara Weatherford, "Comparative Study of Millennials' (Age 20–34 Years) Grip and Lateral Pinch with the Norms," *Journal of Hand Therapy* 29, no. 4 (October 2016): 483–88.

Chapter 6: Sleep Like a Baby

174 **This is true of herbivores:** Jerome M. Siegel, "Clues to the Functions of Mammalian Sleep," *Nature* 437 (2005): 1264–71.

174 **In a detailed study:** Haibin Li and Frank Qian, "Low-Risk Sleep Patterns, Mortality, and Life Expectancy at Age 30 Years: A Prospective Study of 172,321 US Adults," *Journal of the American College of Cardiology* 81, no. Suppl. 8 (March 2023): 1675.

175 **And a British study:** Fengran Tao et al., "Associations of Sleep Duration and Quality with Incident Cardiovascular Disease, Cancer, and Mortality: A Prospective Cohort Study of 407,500 UK Biobank Participants," *Sleep Medicine* 81 (May 2021): 401–9.

175 **One possible explanation:** Luciana Besedovsky, Tanja Lange, and Jan Born, "Sleep and Immune Function," *Pflugers Archiv—European Journal of Physiology* 463 (November 2011): 121–37.

175 **For instance, it lowers:** Karine Spiegel et al., "A Meta-Analysis of the Associations Between Insufficient Sleep Duration and Antibody Response to Vaccination," *Current Biology* 33, no. 5 (March 2023): 998–1005.

175 **Bad sleep patterns:** Janet M. Mullington et al., "Sleep Loss and Inflammation," *Best Practice & Research Clinical Endocrinology & Metabolism* 24, no. 5 (October 2010): 775–84.

175 **In an older meta-analysis:** Francesco P. Cappuccio, et al., "Sleep Duration and All-Cause Mortality: A Systematic Review and Meta-Analysis of Prospective Studies," *Sleep* 33, no. 5 (May 2010): 585–92.

175 **Indeed, for the 172,000 people:** Li and Qian, "Low-Risk Sleep Patterns, Mortality, and Life Expectancy at Age 30 Years."

175 **Studies have found:** A. M. Williamson and Anne-Marie Feyer, "Moderate Sleep Deprivation Produces Impairments in Cognitive and Motor Performance Equivalent to Legally Prescribed Levels of Alcohol Intoxication," *Occupational and Environmental Medicine* 57 (October 2000): 649–55.

176 **Pulling an all-nighter:** Drew Dawson and Kathryn Reid, "Fatigue, Alcohol and Performance Impairment," *Nature* 388, no. 235 (July 1997).

176 **"Sleep deprivation impairs":** "NIOSH Training for Nurses on Shift Work and Long Work Hours," National Institute for Occupational Safety and Health (NIOSH), CDC, last modified March 31, 2020, accessed March 25, 2025.

176 **"moderate, high, and very high":** "NIOSH Training for Nurses," CDC.

176 **Think about the Space Shuttle:** Merrill M. Mitler et al., "Catastrophes,

Sleep, and Public Policy: Consensus Report," *Sleep* 11, no. 1 (January 1988): 100–109.

176 **Too many airplane:** Mitler et al., "Catastrophes, Sleep, and Public Policy."

177 **Participants who reported:** Rebecca Robbins et al., "Examining Sleep Deficiency and Disturbance and Their Risk for Incident Dementia and All-Cause Mortality in Older Adults Across 5 Years in the United States," *Aging* 13, no. 3 (February 2021): 3254–68.

177 **Indeed, seniors who slept:** Robbins et al., "Examining Sleep Deficiency and Disturbance."

177 **Seniors who slept under 7 hours:** Jyri J. Virta et al., "Midlife Sleep Characteristics Associated with Late Life Cognitive Function," *Sleep* 36, no. 10 (October 2013): 1533–41.

177 **Similarly, a recent study:** Linhao Zhang, Charles Geier, Ellen House, and Assaf Oshri, "Latent Default Mode Network Connectivity Patterns: Associations with Sleep Health and Adolescent Psychopathology," *Brain and Behavior* 15, no. 5 (May 2025): e70579.

178 **When asleep, the brain:** Oxana Semyachkina-Glushkovskaya et al., "Brain Waste Removal System and Sleep: Photobiomodulation as an Innovative Strategy for Night Therapy of Brain Diseases," *International Journal of Molecular Sciences* 24, no. 4 (February 2023): 3221.

178 **Namely, sleep facilitates:** Michelle Lampl and Michael L. Johnson, "Infant Growth in Length Follows Prolonged Sleep and Increased Naps," *Sleep* 34, no. 5 (May 2011): 641–50.

178 **While asleep, adenosine:** Carolin Franziska Reichert, Tom Deboer, and Hans-Peter Landolt, "Adenosine, Caffeine, and Sleep-Wake Regulation: State of the Science and Perspectives," special issue, *Journal of Sleep Research* 31, no. 4 (August 2022): e13597

178 **Understanding the role of adenosine:** Christopher Drake et al., "Caffeine Effects on Sleep Taken 0, 3, or 6 Hours Before Going to Bed," *Journal of Clinical Sleep Medicine* 9, no. 11 (November 2013): 1195–1200; Melodee Mograss et al., "The Effects of Napping on Night-Time Sleep in Healthy Young Adults," *Journal of Sleep Research* 31, no. 5 (October 2022): e13578.

180 **And in the spirit:** Laura Nauha et al., "Chronotypes and Objectively Measured Physical Activity and Sedentary Time at Midlife," *Scandinavian Journal of Medicine & Science in Sports* 30, no. 10 (October 2020): 1930–38.

181 **While each person's metabolism:** Institute of Medicine (US) Committee on Military Nutrition Research, "Pharmacology of Caffeine," in *Caffeine for the Sustainment of Mental Task Performance: Formulations for Military Operations*, 2nd ed. (National Academies Press, 2001).

182 **In bed, I read a book:** Anne Mangen, Benete R. Walgenrmo, and Kolbjørn Brønnick, "Reading Linear Texts on Paper Versus Computer Screen: Effects on Reading Comprehension," *International Journal of Educational Research* 58 (January 2013): 61–68.

183 **It improves both REM:** Majd A. Alnawwar et al., "The Effect of Physical Activity on Sleep Quality and Sleep Disorder: A Systematic Review," *Cureus* 15, no. 8 (August 2023): e43595.

183 **A study found that eating more fruits:** Hedda L. Boege, Katherine D. Wilson, Jennifer M. Kilkus, Becky Tucker, Esra Tasali, Marie-Pierre St-Onge, et al., "Higher Daytime Intake of Fruits and Vegetables Predicts Less Disrupted Nighttime Sleep in Younger Adults," *Sleep Health*, June 11, 2025.

183 **Napping after lunch:** Amber Brooks and Leon Lack, "A Brief Afternoon Nap Following Nocturnal Sleep Restriction: Which Nap Duration Is Most Recuperative?," *Sleep* 29, no. 6 (2006): 831–40.

183 **But napping after 2 p.m.:** Janna Mantua and Rebecca M. C. Spencer, "Exploring the Nap Paradox: Are Mid-Day Sleep Bouts a Friend or Foe?," *Sleep Medicine* 37 (September 2017): 88–97.

183 **They might be able:** "Drugstore Sleep Aids May Bring More Risks Than Benefits," Harvard Health Publishing, December 1, 2018, sec. Staying Healthy.

184 **The American Academy of Sleep Medicine:** Michael J. Sateia et al., "Clinical Practice Guideline for the Pharmacologic Treatment of Chronic Insomnia in Adults: An American Academy of Sleep Medicine Clinical Practice Guideline," *Journal of Clinical Sleep Medicine* 13, no. 2 (February 2017): 307–49.

184 **Lots of melatonin pills:** Pieter A. Cohen et al., "Quantity of Melatonin and CBD in Melatonin Gummies Sold in the US," *JAMA* 329, no. 16 (April 2023): 1401–2; Lauren A. E. Erland and Praveen K. Saxena, "Melatonin Natural Health Products and Supplements: Presence of Serotonin and Significant Variability of Melatonin Content," *Journal of Clinical Sleep Medicine* 13, no. 2 (February 2017): 275–81.

184 **The evidence for their effectiveness:** Sateia et al., "Clinical Practice Guideline for the Pharmacologic Treatment of Chronic Insomnia."

184 **"Studies show that sleeping pills":** "Sleeping Pills," Cleveland Clinic, last modified June 22, 2024.

185 **Data suggest that the majority:** Jeffrey Rossman, "Cognitive-Behavioral Therapy for Insomnia: An Effective and Underutilized Treatment for Insomnia," *American Journal of Lifestyle Medicine* 13, no. 6 (August 2019): 544–47.

185 **These problems, though:** Amir Qaseem et al., "Management of Chronic Insomnia Disorder in Adults: A Clinical Practice Guideline From the American College of Physicians," *Annals of Internal Medicine* 165, no. 2 (May 2016): 125–33.

185 **While they have gotten more accurate:** Rebecca Robbins et al., "Accuracy of Three Commercial Wearable Devices for Sleep Tracking in Healthy Adults," *Sensors* 24, no. 20 (October 2024): 6532.

186 **They tend to underestimate deep sleep:** Robbins et al., "Accuracy of Three Commercial Wearable Devices."

186 **In one study, for instance:** Robbins et al., "Accuracy of Three Commercial Wearable Devices."

186 **Overall, at the time:** Robbins et al., "Accuracy of Three Commercial Wearable Devices."

186 **Indeed, this worry:** Kelly Glazer Baron et al., "Orthosomnia: Are Some Patients Taking the Quantified Self Too Far?," *Journal of Clinical Sleep Medicine* 13, no. 2 (February 2017): 351–54.

186 **"The most accurate measure of good sleep":** William Lu, "The Real Deal on Sleep Tracking: Is It Worth Your Time?," *Dreem Health* (blog), last modified November 3, 2024.

Afterword: Be a Mensch

189 **"Family is for me":** Therese Murray, "Family Is the Key to a Long Life, Say Five Supercentenarians from Around Australia," *The Senior*, September 24, 2021.

189 **"Friends, a good cigar":** Associated Press, "Christian Mortensen, 115, Among Oldest," *New York Times*, May 3, 1998, sec. U.S.
189 **"all participants, regarding of their living":** Wai-Ching Paul Wong et al., "The Well-Being of Community-Dwelling near-Centenarians and Centenarians in Hong Kong a Qualitative Study," *BMC Geriatrics* 14, no. 63 (May 2014).
189 **"were highly social":** Ed Diener and Martin E. P. Seligman, "Very Happy People," *Psychological Science* 13, no. 1 (January 2002): 81–84.
189 **Many Latin American countries:** Mariangela Rodriguez, "The Well-Being Paradox in Latin America: What Should Be Protected and What Can Be Learned," MAPP Magazine, July 10, 2024; Mariano Rojas, "The Joint Enjoyment of Life. Explaining High Happiness in Latin America," *Journal of Happiness Studies* 25, no. 100 (2024); Jan-Emmanuel De Neve, Andrew Dugan, Micah Kaats, and Alberto Prati, "Sharing Meals with Others: How Sharing Meals Supports Happiness and Social Connections," World Happiness Report 2025, chap. 3.
191 **After all, he lived:** J. David Hacker, "Decennial Life Tables for the White Population of the United States, 1790–1900," *Historical Methods* 43, no. 2 (April 2010): 45–79.
192 **Or as he might summarize:** H. W. Brands, *The First American: The Life and Times of Benjamin Franklin* (Doubleday, 2000).
192 **All the data show:** Lara B. Aknin and Ashley V. Whillans, "Helping and Happiness: A Review and Guide for Public Policy," *Social Issues and Policy Review* 15, no. 1 (2021): 3–34.
193 **Franklin would have advised:** Benjamin Franklin, *Benjamin Franklin's Autobiography: A Norton Critical Edition,* ed. Joyce E. Chaplin (W. W. Norton, 2012).